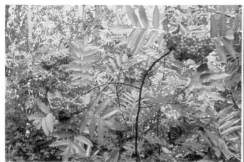

Mountain Ash, *p. 124*
Sorbus spp.

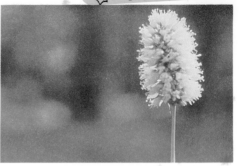

Bistort, *p. 33*
Polygonium bistordoides

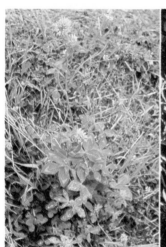

Red Clover, *p. 146*
Trifolium spp.

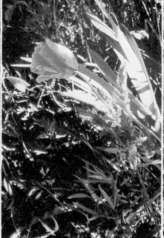

California Poppy, *p. 48*
Eschoscholtzia californica

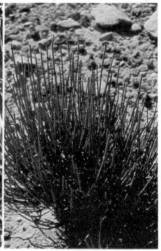

Mormon Tea, *p. 122*
Ephedra spp.

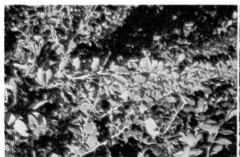

Barberry, *p. 28*
Berberis vulgaris

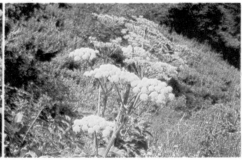

Cow Parsnip, *p. 64*
Heracleum spp.

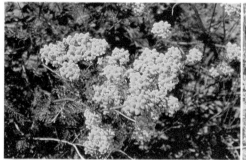

Yarrow, *p. 181*
Achillea millefolium

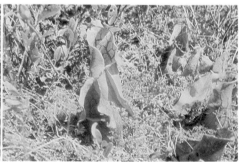

Pitcher Plant, *p. 140*
Sarracenia spp.

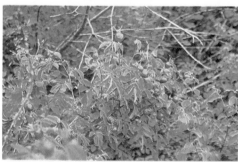

Rose Hips, *p. 150*
Rosa spp.

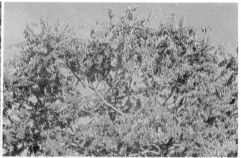

Sumac, p. 165
Rhus spp.

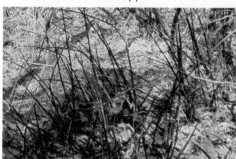

Horsetails, *p. 92*
Equisetum spp.

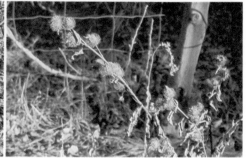

Burdock, *p. 46*
Lappa

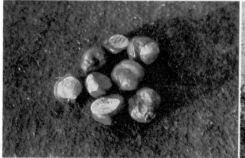

Horse Chestnuts, *p. 90*
Aesculus hippocastanum

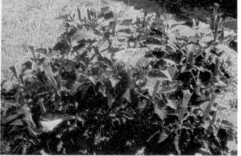

Jimson Weed, *p. 101*
Datura stramonium

Herbal Medications

David G. Spoerke, Jr.

Associate Clinical Professor of Clinical Pharmacy
University of Utah College of Pharmacy
Managing Director
Intermountain Regional Poison Control Center

Published by
Woodbridge Press Publishing Company
Santa Barbara, California 93111

Please Note: The information in this book is presented as a matter of general interest only. It is not in any way a prescription for any specific person or condition. It consists of the best information available to the author through his research of the scientific literature and personal observation. Other research and observation may produce differing information and opinions. In every case, where a specific health problem or concern exists, competent professional advice should be sought.

Published by
Woodbridge Press Publishing Company
Post Office Box 6189
Santa Barbara, California 93111

Copyright © 1980 by David G. Spoerke, Jr.

Photographs by the author.

Printed in the United States of America
Published simultaneously in Canada

Library of Congress Cataloging in Publication Data

Spoerke, David G
  Herbal medications.

  Bibliography: p.
  Includes index.
  1. Herbs—Therapeutic use. 2. Medicinal Plants.
I. Title. [DNLM: 1. Herbalism. 2. Herbs. WB925
S762h]
RM666.H33S64   615'.321   80-17551
ISBN 0-912800-72-8

To Betsy—Who taught me to appreciate what nature has given us, but to temper this knowledge with judgment.

Acknowledgments

This text was edited by Susan E. Spoerke, M.D., Salt Lake City, Utah; and Nancy Davidson of Santa Barbara, California.

A special thanks to Sheila Banks for her many hours of secretarial assistance and advice.

Contents

Introduction

This is a book concerning plants and how they are used to treat a variety of human illnesses and diseases. There is a growing number of people who are turning to "natural" means of health care, and this frequently means the use of herbs and health foods. Some of these people say that herbal medicines are the only true means of obtaining "natural" health. They pit themselves against those who think that all herbal medication is quackery and that the only safe, effective drugs are those produced by the pharmaceutical industry. The truth, of course, lies between these two extremes. Plants have many times been the original source of many drugs and the drug companies still cultivate some species to provide either raw material or actual drugs. Many of nature's remedies have been changed, however, to make them more potent, more specific, or easier to use. Whether you see this as good or bad depends on your point of view.

This book will present the uses of many of these herbs in the light of what is known about their constituents and activity. In fact, many of the herbs used today have had little pharmacologic testing; information concerning their actions and effectiveness is lacking. Even when the chemicals are known, there are often only minimal tests to date to shed light on their activity. Such testing is costly, and much of the time would not result in a drug more "salable" than one currently on the market. The major areas of conflicts between the above two groups arise because of this inability

7

to prove the actions of various herbs. Just because an herb has been used for hundreds of years does not mean that it has any actual pharmacologic value, or that it has greater value than an already existing agent. Conversely, just because no pharmacologic activity can be found does not necessarily mean that the herb is useless. Actually, most of that activity is often overstated. This text aims to clarify some of the claims made for various herbs. If no basis in fact can be found for the use of a particular herb, it will be so stated. If there is a definite reason for its activity, this will be mentioned.

Another major area of concern for those who oppose the widespread use of herbs is the belief that herbs are harmless. Some think that although herbs may be helpful, they cannot be harmful. This assumption is, of course, not true. In fact, those that have enough pharmacologic activity to be useful are often the very ones to pose the greatest hazards. Biological activity is a two-edged sword, and this should not be forgotten. Herb use may become hazardous for several reasons. For one thing, the quantity of active herb in a preparation is often extremely variable. This may be the result of an improperly prepared product, biological variation in the plant itself, choice of plant part used, or out-and-out fraud on the part of the seller. This variability can be dangerous if a user must have a certain dose every day to maintain his condition. Another danger is the use of herbs to treat illnesses for which they have no activity, or for which they may be contraindicated. For example, the use of cayenne pepper to treat a stomach ulcer is not only not useful, but will aggravate the condition. Similarly, the slight expectorant action of catnip is unlikely to be of significant aid in treating a bacterial pneumonia. In cases like the latter, the herb causes harm by delaying treatment with more effective agents.

Each herb monograph is divided into a number of sections. The first of these states some of the names given to each herb. A number of common names are given as well as the Latin genus and species names. Although use of common names may be simpler, a single name is often used for a number of different herbs, leading to confusion in identification. In comparing or evaluating herbs, always note the genus and species names to be sure of which herb is meant.

The second section lists the *known* principles contained in the herb. *Known* principles are stressed since many herbs have had only minimal chemical analysis. This section will be most useful to physicians, pharmacists, nurses, and those who have an interest in medicinal chemistry. It can also be of use in making comparisons of actions by looking at common active ingredients.

Section three discusses the suggested mechanisms of action for each plant. Not all monographs are equally detailed because of the wide variability in original research. Next in the monograph is a discussion of the alleged uses for each plant. Occasionally evaluations are made as to whether these professed effects have any basis in fact. Such suggested uses range from treatment of disease to avoidance of demons. The pharmacology of demon-warding is not well known or understood by modern science, so little comment will be made concerning these claims.

The fifth area deals with the potential of the plant to cause adverse effects or poisonings. Again, although information is sadly lacking with many of these herbs, an attempt is made to evaluate each herb's potential for harm if misused.

The next section will contain any other specific comments regarding the herb. These may range from the history of the plant to a suggested mechanism of action.

The last section deals with the references used to prepare the monograph. Whenever possible statements made in the text have been referenced. The reference list is available at the end of the text and is keyed to the numbers found in the monographs.

Information presented in this format should interest a wide variety of individuals. If one's area is toxicology, medicinal chemistry, or home treatment, this guide should provide useful information. Those with specific interests need read only the sections pertaining to their interests. If more general information is desired, it should be available elsewhere in the monograph.

Glossary of Terms

Abortifacient—An agent that induces abortions.

Acids—Compounds often found in plant tissues, especially fruits, which have astringency as a common property.

Active Principle—The chemical component of a crude drug that has a therapeutic effect.

Adulterant—A substance used to make corrupt or impure (by mixing).

Alkaloid—Alkaloids are extremely difficult to define, since they do not represent a homogenous group of compounds, either from chemical, biological, or physiological points of view. Except that all are organic nitrogenous compounds, reservations must be applied to any general definition. Alkaloids are usually classified according to the nature of the basic chemical structures from which they are derived. Most alkaloids are biologically active if the quantity administered is sufficient.

Allergen—A substance capable of inducing an allergy or a specific susceptibility.

Amenorrhea—The absence or abnormal stoppage of the menses.

Anesthetic—A drug or chemical agent used to abolish the sensation of pain.

Anthelmintic—An agent that is destructive to worms.

Antibacterial—A substance that destroys bacteria or suppresses their growth or reproduction.

11

Anticoagulant—Any substance that suppresses, delays, or cancels coagulation of the blood.

Antimitotic—Any substance that inhibits or prevents cell division.

Antineoplastic—Inhibiting or preventing the growth of neoplasms (cancers).

Antipyretic—An agent that will reduce or cancel fevers.

Antiseptic—Any substance that will inhibit the growth and development of microorganisms without necessarily destroying them.

Antispasmodic—Any agent that relieves the spasm of either skeletal or smooth muscle.

Aperitive—A substance that will stimulate the appetite.

Aphrodisiac—Any substance that arouses the sexual instinct.

Astringent—A substance that shrinks tissues and prevents the secretions of fluids.

Aromatic—A medicinal substance with a spicy fragrance and stimulant qualities.

Bitter—A medicinal agent that has a bitter taste. Its action is usually local (as opposed to systemic) and is exerted in the gastrointestinal tract. Bitters are used as a tonic or appetizer.

Bronchitis—Any inflammation of the bronchi.

Bulb—A modified plant bud with scaly leaves that occurs beneath the soil.

Cardiac arrhythmias—Any abnormal heart rate or rhythm.

Carminative—An agent that aids in expelling gas from the gastrointestinal tract so as to relieve colic or griping.

Cathartic—A strong laxative.

Central Nervous System Depressant (CNS depressant)—Any

agent that by acting on the brain will cause drowsiness or coma.

Conjunctivitis—Inflammation of the front or outer membrane of the eye.

Colic—Acute abdominal pain.

Counterirritant—An agent that causes an irritation that is intended to relieve another irritation.

Cyanogenic Glycoside—A glycoside that will release cyanide in the intestines.

Cystitis—Inflammation of the bladder.

Decoction—An extract of a crude drug obtained by boiling the agent in water.

Dehiscent—This describes a fruit that splits open when ripe.

Demonic—An agent that is meant to repel or destroy a demon.

Demulcent—A usually mucilaginous or oily substance capable of serving as protection for abraded tissues.

Dermatitis—Any of a number of various skin irritations or inflammations.

Diaphoretic—A substance for increasing perspiration.

Diuretic—A substance that helps the body to dispose of water by increasing the amount of urine produced.

Drupe—A fleshy fruit with a hard stone, such as a peach.

Dysentery—A term given to a number of disorders marked by inflammation of the intestines, especially of the colon, and attended by pain in the abdomen, tenesmus, and frequent stools containing blood and/or mucus.

Dyspepsia—An impairment in the powers or function of digestion.

Eclectic Physician—A physician who professes to select what is best from all systems of medicine.

Eczema—An inflammatory disease of the skin.

Emetic—A substance that causes vomiting.

Emmenagogue—A substance that brings on menstruation.

Emollient—Any agent that softens or sooothes.

Enema—A liquid preparation introduced into the rectum.

Eupeptic—A substance that promotes good digestion.

Essential Oils—See volatile oil.

Expectorant—An agent that tends to decrease the viscosity and promote the discharge of mucus from the respiratory tract.

Extract—An extract is prepared by leaving a plant in any solvent for a time, then allowing the solution to evaporate. This concentrate is called an extract. It may be a fluid extract, or if greater evaporation is allowed, a soft extract. In some cases all the solvent is evaporated, leaving a dry extract that may be powdered.

Flatulence—A distention of the stomach or intestines by air or other gases.

Fixed Oil—(Lipids, fats, waxes) These are esters of long chain fatty acids and alcohols. Fixed oils and fats differ only in the melting points and are quite bland. They often are seed oils such as linseed or flaxseed oil.

Fluid Extract—An alcoholic preparation of a drug of plant origin. Fluid extracts usually contain one gram of dry drug in each milliliter.

Gastroenteritis—Inflammation of the stomach and intestines, characterized by pain, nausea, and diarrhea.

Gastrointestinal—Pertaining to the region of the stomach or intestines.

Gingivitis—Any inflammation of the gums.

Glycosides—These yield, upon hydrolysis, one or more

sugars among the products of hydrolysis. The glycosides are sugar ethers, in which the nonsugar component is aglycone, and the sugar portion is glycone. Glycosides contribute to almost every therapeutic class.

Griping—Intestinal cramping.

Gums—Gums are natural plant hydrocolloids that are classified as polysaccharides or salts of polysaccharides. They are translucent, amorphous substances produced by plants as protection after injury. Gums are differentiated from mucilages on the basis that gums readily dissolve in water and mucilages do not dissolve. Mucilages also tend to be physiological products and gums are pathological products. Both gums and mucilages are generally considered decomposition products of cellulose.

Hallucinogen—An agent that produces a sense perception not founded on objective reality.

Hemolysis—The breaking or destruction of red blood cells.

Hemorrhages—Various types of bleeding.

Hemostatic—Any substance that will prevent bleeding or promotes clotting of blood.

Herb—A plant or plant part valued for its medicinal, savory, or aromatic qualities.

Homeopathy—A system of therapeutics founded by Samuel Hahnemann, in which diseases are treated by drugs that are capable of producing, in healthy persons, symptoms like those of the disease to be treated. Drugs are usually administered in small doses in this type of therapy.

Humectant—A moistening or diluent substance.

Indehiscent—Fruits that remain closed upon reaching maturity.

Inflorescence—The flowerhead of a plant.

Infusion—The product of the process of steeping a drug

for the extraction of its medicinal properties.

Lactagogue—An agent that increases the flow of milk.

Latex—A milky juice produced by certain plants.

Larvacide—Any substance known to kill larvae.

Laxative—A substance that encourages defecation.

Maceration—The softening of a solid by soaking. Generally, cold-water extract of a plant.

Mitogen—An agent that causes or induces cell division.

Mucilage—A gelatinous substance that contains proteins and polysaccharides and is similar to plant gums. (See gums.)

Narcotic—Any agent that produces insensibility or stupor.

Oleoresin—Resins and volatile oils in a homogenous mixture.

Peduncle—A stalk attached to a flower.

Peristalsis—A wave of contractions produced by both the longitudinal and circular muscles to propel contents along the tube, especially the alimentary canal.

Pharmacognosy—The study of the biology, chemistry, and pharmacology of plant drugs, herbs, and spices.

Pharmacology—The study of the actions of chemicals and drugs in the body.

Pharyngitis—Any inflammation of the throat.

Photosensitization—The process by which a substance or organism becomes sensitive to light.

Poultice—A soft, moist mass applied hot to a surface for the purpose of applying heat and moisture. It occasionally acts as a means of applying medication.

Powder—Finely divided sieved or sifted dry particles.

Psoriasis—A chronic recurrent skin disease.

Pulmonary—Anything concerning the lungs.

Purgative—Any powerful laxative.

Pyorrhea—A discharge of pus from the gums or teeth.

Renal—Referring to the kidneys.

Resin—Resins are amorphous products of a complex chemical nature. Physically they are usually hard, transparent, or translucent, and upon heating, soften and melt. Chemically, they are complex mixtures of acid resins, resin alcohols, resinotannols, esters, and resenes. These agents are frequently pharmacologically active and often associated with negative pharmacological effects.

Rhizome—A somewhat elongate, usually horizontal subterranean plant stem that is thickened by deposits of reserve food materials. It produces shoots above the roots and is distinguished from the true root in possessing buds, nodes, and usually scaled-like leaves.

Roots—The underground portion of a plant that never bears leaves or reproductive organs and serves to absorb salts and solutions.

Rubefacient—An agent that reddens the skin by producing active or passive increases of blood to the skin.

Saponin—Any of various surfactant glycosides, mostly toxic, that occur in plants, and are characterized by properties of producing soapy lather.

Scrofula—Tuberculosis of the lymphatic glands and sometimes of bones and joint surfaces, which usually produces marked irregular superficial ulcers.

Sepal—A segment of the calyx, the external green or leafy part of flowers.

Spasmolytic—Any agent that decreases spasms. See antispasmodic.

Stimulant—A substance that stimulates activities of the body.

Stomachic—An agent that promotes activity of the stomach.

Stomatitis—Any inflammation of the mouth.

Tannins—Noncrystalline chemicals, which with water form colloidal solutions possessing an acid reaction and a "puckering" taste. They precipitate solutions of proteins and alkaloids. Chemically, tannins are complex mixtures of polyphenols. Most tannins, when hydrolyzed, yield simple polyhydroic phenols such as gallic, proto-catechuic, and ellatic acids. One property all tannins have in common is that they give a blue, green, or black color to anything that contains iron.

Tenesmus—Any ineffectual and painful straining at stool or in urination.

Terpenes—Isomeric hydrocarbons having a molecular formula $C_{10}H_{16}$. Most volatile oils consist primarily of terpenes.

Therapeutics—A branch of medicine associated with the use of remedies and the treatment of diseases.

Tincture—A solution of chemicals in a highly alcoholic solvent made by simple solution or by methods described in USP or NF.

Tonic—The term formally used for a class of medicinal preparations believed to have the power of restoring normal tone to tissues.

Toxicity—The quality of being poisonous.

Umbel—An umbrella-shaped inflorescence.

Vasodilatation—A dilating of blood vessels.

Vermifuge—An agent that destroys or expels worms or intestinal animal parasites.

Volatile Oil—Odorous principles found in various plants, which, because they evaporate at ordinary temperatures, are called etheral or essential oils. Chemical constituents of volatile oils may be divided into two classes —the terpene derivative and aromatic compounds.

Herbal Medications

Agave
(*Agave lecheguilla* and other species)

Known Principles: Agave contains steroidal sapogenins and a photosensitizing pigment.

Mode of Action: The actions of saponins are seldom specific, but in general, they are irritant substances that produce cellular damage, tissue permeability changes, and erythrocyte hemolysis. Saponins may be gastric irritants and visceral vasodilators as well. Absorption through intact mucous membranes is poor; therefore, systemic hormone therapy or as immunosuppressives. These include hecogenin, manogenin, and gitogenin.

Alleged Uses: Agave parts are used for a number of non-medicinal purposes. These include the sap as a nutrient syrup and the fibers as rope. The root and leaves have sometimes been recommended to relieve toothache. *Agave parryi* is used to make mescal, an alcoholic beverage, and is said to be edible and wholesome.

Toxicity: Symptoms of poisoning include nausea, vomiting, diarrhea, visceral vasodilatation, and hemorrhage. It has also caused various types of dermatitis, liver damage, and photosensitization. It has sometimes been recommended as an abortifacient. The leaves have poisoned range animals, causing 30% morbidity in severe outbreaks.

Comments: Agave contains several types of plant steroids that have been investigated for possible uses in either

19

hormone therapy or as immunosuppressives. These include hecogenin, manogenin, and gitogenin.

References: 7, 8, 16, 17, 34

Alfalfa
(*Medicago sativa*)

Known Principles: Alfalfa contains vitamins A, B, K, and D.

Mode of Action: Alfalfa is most commonly used as a dietary supplement for its high protein and vitamin content. There is no available evidence to support its use as an antiarthritis agent.

Alleged Uses: The young leaves and flowering tops are ground up and taken as compressed tablets or capsules. Occasionally the above-ground portion is made into a tea. Alfalfa has been recommended as a treatment for hemorrhage, probably due to its Vitamin K content. Some claim it is of aid in treatment of arthritis.

Toxicity: There is no evidence to indicate that alfalfa presents a toxic hazard.

References: 2, 10, 13

Allspice (Pimenta)
(*Pimenta officinalis*)

Known Principles: Allspice berries contain 1–4% of a volatile oil, a small amount of resin, tannic acid, and an acrid fixed oil. The volatile oil is 60–75% eugenol, but also contains cineole, levophellandrene, caryophyllene, eugenol methyl ether, and palmitic acid.

Mode of Action: Most activity comes from the volatile oil eugenol. The herb has mucous membrane irritant properties and is a carminative.

Alleged Uses: Pimenta is an aromatic carminative and flavor. Besides its use in cosmetics and toothpaste, it is used as an aromatic spice in foods. Its odor is supposed to smell like a mixture of cloves, cinnamon and nutmeg. Medically, allspice is used as an adjuvant to tonics and purgatives, as well as a carminative and antidiarrheal.

Toxicity: Although there are no reports of allspice poisoning, there have been overdoses of eugenol. Care should be taken when using the oil, as amounts in excess of 5 ml may cause nausea, vomiting, CNS depression and/or convulsions.

References: 1, 2, 16, 17, 24

Aloe
(*Aloe barbadensis, A. vera, A. officinalis*)
(Burn Plant)

Known Principles: The purgative properties are probably due to barbaloin (5–30%), socaloin (7.5–10%), capaloin (4.5–9%). Some species may also contain isobarbaloin and beta-barbaloin. Aloe vera usually does not contain barbaloin, the most important of the ingredients. All of the above are aloe-emodin combinations with D-arabinose. There is also a resinoltannol (16-63%) that appears to play an important role.

Mode of Action: The aloe-emodin are cathartics that stimulate peristalsis, especially in the lower bowel. They are even more irritating than cascara sagrada or senna. Action usually starts 12-18 hours post ingestion. The presence of bile in the gut is very important for this agent's action. Although some studies have shown aloe to be effective against several microorganisms, especially

Pseudomonas aeruginosa, the inhibitory agent is either not always present or very unstable, since other studies are contradictory. Even though several chemical investigations have been done, none of the organic structures isolated have significance in the healing process.

Alleged Uses: Aloe has been recommended for many uses, including aid to amenorrhea, sexual enhancement, increased development of mammary glands, and external application to the forehead to relieve headache. The two uses that have persisted in folk medicine the longest are as a burn treatment and a laxative. There is good reason for its use as a laxative, but much experience is still needed to substantiate its use in burns. Studies in 1935, 1937, and 1939 showed an increased healing when both roentgen and thermal burns were treated with aloe. Only the milky exudate is used for treatment, and it must not be dried before use or it loses its effectiveness. Effective life of an application is 1–2 hours, and it turns from light green to a dark gummy mass, and should be removed.

Toxicity: External application appears to be relatively harmless. Minor skin irritation is possible. Internally one may experience cramps, nausea, vomiting, or diarrhea. The urine may be colored red, and kidney inflammation may occur if taken chronically.

Comments: The product is contraindicated in conditions where small bowel irritation would create a problem. Since it clears only the lower bowel, it is not useful as a presurgery cathartic. Studies still need to be done to discover the nature of any healing aid in aloe. There is too much evidence to ignore this property, but as yet the nature of any such aid is unknown.

References: 2, 17, 32, 33

Alum Root
(Heuchera spp.) (American Sanicle)

Known Principles: Alum root contains 9.3–20% tannins.

Mode of Action: The tannins are protein precipitants and astringents.

Alleged Uses: The rhizomes of this plant were used by the Nevada and Utah Indians for heart disease and used externally and internally as an astringent. It has a strong, styptic taste.

Toxicity: Tannins are gastric irritants and may cause kidney and liver failure. One gram of tannic acid has been tolerated without serious symptoms—this would be 5-10 gms of the plant material. Amounts greater than this may present a hazard.

References: 1, 17

American Dogwood
(Cornus florida)

Known Principles: One 1836 study found cornin (a glycoside), while another study in 1939 found betulic acid. Cornin has also been called verbenalin and is the iridoid glycoside found in wild hyssop.

Mode of Action: Cornin is a very bitter astringent iridoid glycoside. It has possible external antibacterial action. It also has cathartic action at 110 mg per kilogram, causing catharsis in approximately one hour. It has an action on the uterus similar to ergot and is a weak parasympathomimetic. It does not appear to have any antipyretic action.

Alleged Uses: American dogwood has been recommended as a quinine substitute. The bark is the portion of the plant used for treatment of fevers. The normal dose recommended is 2–4 ml of the fluid extract.

Toxicity: There is little data concerning the American dogwood, but it does appear that the plant may cause dermatitis. Verbenalin does have low toxicity compared to other members of the iridoid glycoside group.

References: 3, 17, 36, 39

Angelica
(*Angelica archangelica* and other species)

Known Principles: Fruits contain about 1% of a volatile oil, the roots around 0.3–1%. There is also angelic acid, resin, and some starch.

Mode of Action: The irritant action of the volatile oil gives it some expectorant and diaphoretic properties.

Alleged Uses: The seeds and roots have primarily been used as an aromatic in flatulent colic and as a domestic diaphoretic and diuretic. The seeds are supposed to contain antimalarial activity, but this has not been substantiated. Dose of the seed or root is 1-2 gms.

Toxicity: No toxic ingestions have been reported.

Comments: This herb was officially listed in the British Pharmacopeia in 1934.

References: 1, 17

Anise
(*Pimpinella anisum*)

Known Principles: Anise contains 1–3% of a volatile oil (which is 80–90% anethole), 3–4% of a fixed oil, and some calcium oxalate.

Mode of Action: This herb is a stimulant aromatic and a carminative. It possesses diuretic and diaphoretic properties. As an expectorant, it may act directly on the secretory cells of the respiratory tract.

Alleged Uses: Medically, anise is used internally to decrease flatulence and colic. Externally it has been applied to kill body lice. It is also used extensively as a flavoring agent. The normal dose of the oil is 0.2–0.3 ml.

Toxicity: Anise itself is low in toxicity. The oil distilled from the herb may cause some skin irritation, nausea, vomiting, seizures, or pulmonary edema. As little as 1–5 ml may cause symptoms.

References: 2, 3, 10, 17

Asafetida
(*Ferula assafoetida, F. foetida*) (Devil's Dung)

Known Principles: Asafetida contains 25% gum, 3–17% volatile oil, 40–60% resin, and a number of other trace constituents. The resin, consisting of esters of asaresinotannol and ferulic acid, upon dry distillation yields the compound umbelliferone. The volatile oil contains diallyl disulfide, allyl propyl disulfide, and probably diallyltrisulfide, pinene, cadinene, and vanillin.

Mode of Action: The volatile oil in asafetida has been used for its carminative and expectorant properties in treating flatulence and bronchitis. The volatile oil is eliminated by way of the lungs; therefore the drug has been used as a stimulant expectorant in chronic bronchitis, whooping cough, and asthma. Although it is absorbed from the intestinal tract, there appears to be little evidence that it has any distinct action. A human volunteer once took ½ ounce at one time without effects other than a local action.

Alleged Uses: Asafetida is a gum-resin obtained as an exudate of the cut rhizomes and roots of the plants. It is usually found in the form of grayish-white or yellowish waxy tears with a garlic-like odor and bitter, acrid taste. Nonmedically, it is used as a condiment, flavor, and ingredient in Worcestershire sauce, and a 2% solution as a repellent for dogs, cats, and other animals. Medically it is primarily administered as an expectorant for chronic cough or colic. In small infants, it is sometimes administered rectally. It has also found some uses as a laxative. Asafetida has formerly been recommended for its effect in nerve disorders, but this effect is now thought to be due to the psychological effect of administering a product with such a disagreeable odor and taste. The normal dose of the herb is 300 mg to 1 gm.

Toxicity: There are few cases of toxic exposures to this herb. One reference indicates there may be some skin rashes with prolonged contact.

Comments: Asafetida was introduced to European medicine by Arabian physicians.

References: 1, 2, 9, 16, 17, 29

Bachelor's Buttons
(*Chrysanthemum parthenium*) (Feverfew)

Known Principles: References indicate that feverfew probably contains pyrethrins, and most likely has two other compounds called parthenolide and santamarin.

Mode of Action: The information concerning the pharmacologic effect of bachelor's buttons is extremely limited. The pyrethrins, if present, are probably insecticidal. There also appears to be some mucous membrane effect that could cause some diaphoresis and produce an expectorant action.

Alleged Uses: The alleged uses of bachelor's buttons are many and varied. The leaves have been recommended to treat bad colds, indigestion, and diarrhea, and to ease parturition and decrease edema. Dried flowers have been used to treat intestinal worms, to induce menstrual flow, and even to bring about abortion. It is also used as an appetite stimulant, a carminative, and as an active bitter.

Toxicity: There is no conclusive data on the toxicity of bachelor's buttons. If it does contain pyrethrin, sensitivity (allergic) reactions may occur.

Comments: Bachelor's buttons has little approved efficacy, especially for its many varied uses. Its actual therapeutic effects are still very much in doubt. Bachelor's buttons is a common name for several plants. Please check the genus and species names when comparing.

References: 36, 39, 40, 41

Barberry
(Berberis vulgaris)

Known Principles: Barberry contains eight different alkaloids: oxycanthine, berbamine, berberine, palmatine, jatrorrhizine, columbamine, berberrubine, and hydrastine. The first three are in the highest concentration and therefore are the most pharmacologically important.

Mode of Action: Berberine in animals produces vasodilatation by direct action and decreases heart rate through vagal stimulation. Other studies indicate that berberine has a distinct stimulant effect on the myocardium in low doses. However, higher doses depress the myocardium. High doses also depress respiration, stimulate intestinal smooth muscle, and reduce bronchial constriction. Berberine also has a mild anesthetic action on mucous membranes and has been noted to inhibit cultures of *Leishmania tropica* at a dilution of 1:80,000 (1.3% of the concentration of quinine needed). Hydrastine may produce a decrease in intestinal smooth muscle tone.

Alleged Uses: Various parts of the plant are used. The fruit is made into jelly, and the roots into a wool dye and a medicine. The powdered bark is taken 3–4 times daily. Berberine's astringent properties may have been useful in treating diarrhea, while its bitterness may cause increased gastric secretions (an aid in dyspepsia).

Toxicity: Children eat berries with little harm; the roots may give symptoms of mucous membrane irritation, nausea, vomiting, and in large amounts, hypotension, heart failure, and convulsions.

Comments: Claims of the efficacy of this agent are apparently based upon folklore and limited laboratory experimentation.

References: 1, 3, 4, 5, 6, 7, 9, 10, 13, 16, 17, 18

Barley
(Hordeum distichon, Hordeum spp.)

Known Principles: Barley contains primarily nutrients. These include 60–68% starch, 8–17% pentosans, 7–14% nitrogenous substances, 4–5% cellulose, 1.5–2.5% sucrose, 4% lignin, some pectin, invert sugar, ash, and malt. Besides these nutrients, it also contains hordein, a protein related to gliadin, and the alkaloid hordenine, which is related to ephedrine, mescaline, and sparteine.

Mode of Action: The material is mucilaginous, so it has some demulcent properties. It is also a nutrient rich in mineral salts. The alkaloid does not seem to produce hallucinations even though it is related to similar agents.

Alleged Uses: Barley is primarily used as a "restorative" and demulcent for stomach and intestinal irritations.

Toxicity: There appears to be little toxic change from the plant itself. Barley infested with fungus has caused animal poisonings.

Comments: Used extensively in brewing and beverage industries.

References: 1, 2, 17 36

Bayberry
(Myrica cerifera)

Known Principles: The bark of the root contains an acrid and astringent resin. The plant also contains tannic and gallic acids and the palmitin-containing myricic wax. The acrid substance called myricinic acid, which seems to be related to saponins, may also be found.

Mode of Action: Bayberry does have some astringency due to both the resin as well as the saponinic compound myricinic acid. This saponin is especially irritating and may cause vomiting.

Alleged Uses: Bayberry is used internally as an astringent and emetic. Externally it has been applied to ulcers. It is commonly added to other herbals for use against the common cold as well as an aid in the treatment of diarrhea and jaundice. The bark of the root has been used on decoctions for "spongy" gums. Bayberry wax is frequently used in manufacturing of cosmetics, pharmaceuticals, and in candle making.

Toxicity: There is no evidence that therapeutic amounts of bayberry are harmful.

References: 2, 3, 16, 17

Bearberry
(*Arctostaphylos* spp.) (Uva-ursi)

Known Principles: Bearberry contains arbutin (known also as ursin), which hydrolyzes in gastric fluid to form hydroquinolone in dextrose. Berries contain about 10% arbutin, 6% tannins, a volatile oil, quercetin, ericolin, gallic acid, malic acid, and ursolic acid.

Mode of Action: This herb's primary pharmacologic action is most likely due to the hydroquinolone. Hydroquinolone is primarily effective in alkaline urine of where it exerts a mild astringent and antiseptic action. The urine is often green when uva-ursi is used. Ursolic acid (urson) and isoquercetin have also been isolated from the plant. These agents are strong diuretics in a 1:100,000 dilution.

Alleged Uses: A solution is prepared by boiling bruised leaves in water for 15 minutes. The leaves also have been smoked. Bearberry's primary uses are as a diuretic, astringent, and mild central nervous system depressant. It is also a vehicle for other medications.

Toxicity: The ingestion of large amounts would be expected to produce mild central nervous system depression, nausea, tinnitus, and some respiratory embarrassment. This herb is relatively safe, and no symptoms are expected in quantities generally available.

References: 1, 3, 4, 5, 6, 9, 12, 14, 17

Birch
(*Betula alba, B. lenta*)

Known Principles: Leaves and shoots secrete a resin, which when combined with alkali is said to create a laxative substance. The bark contains 10–14% betulin (a dihydric alcohol). When made into birch bark tar, the tar contains creosol, traces of phenols, creosote, and guaiacol. *Betula lenta* bark contains significant amounts of methyl salicylate.

Mode of Action: The methyl salicylate of *B. lenta* may be used as a counterirritant in treating rheumatism. It also has some analgesic properties. The betulin has unknown pharmacologic properties.

Alleged Uses: The leaves have an agreeable, aromatic odor and have been used as an infusion for rheumatism and dropsy. Both the leaves and the bark have a bitter taste. The bark has been used as an astringent, while birch has found use in treatment for various types of skin disorders.

Toxicity: There does not appear to be enough pharmacologic activity associated with the betulin to make
overdose a hazard. One could become poisoned on the
methyl salicylate in *B. lenta* bark, or have significant der-
mal irritation due to the phenolic components of the
birch bark tar.

References: 1, 17

Birthroot
(Trillium erectum, T. pendulum) (Bethroot)

Known Principles: *Trillium* species are said to contain a volatile oil, a fixed oil, tannic acid, the saponin trillarin (a
diglycoside of diosgenin), a glycoside resembling convallamarin, a crystalline acid, a resin, and considerable
starch.

Mode of Action: Pharmacologic studies on this plant are
sorely lacking. The saponin could have significant mucous membrane irritation and cause severe gastrointestinal distress. The convallamarin-like glycoside could
cause some heart activity as well.

Alleged Uses: The Southeastern Indians used this plant as an
aphrodisiac. In the 1800s, it was commonly used to decrease heart palpitations, control skin infections, and stop
hemorrhages. The name "birthroot" comes about because the pioneers used it for the hemorrhages after
parturition. From this use it has been recommended for
treatment of various other uterine disorders such as me-
trorrhagia and menorrhagia. *Trillium* has found some use
as an astringent, expectorant, and externally as an astringent poultice.

Toxicity: There have been no reports of poisoning with *trillium*, but considering the known principles, the possibility does exist. Perhaps the plant has low activity.

Comments: In 1938 a study was done on trillarin and trillium root. All samples studied were physiologically inert.

References: 2, 6, 10, 17, 39

Bistort
(Polygonum bistorta) (Snakeweed)

Known Principles: This plant contains up to 20% tannins.

Mode of Action: Tannins are protein precipitants and astringents.

Alleged Uses: The root (1.3–2 gms) is most often used as an astringent gargle, treatment for hemorrhages, and an emetic. The roots are sometimes mixed equally with *Anacyclus pyrethrum* and alum, then beaten into a paste that is placed in or beside carious teeth.

Toxicity: Little is available on its toxicity, but 20% tannins is a significant concentration. Large or frequent doses could cause vomiting, gastritis, or kidney damage.

References: 10, 17

Bitter Root
(Apocynum androsaemifolium)
(Wild Ipecac, Dogbane, Rheumatism Weed)

Known Principles: Bitter root contains the impure amorphous solids apocynein and apocynin. These are most likely saponins. The aglycone of the glycosides apocynamarin is called cymarin. Cymarin is closely related to glycosides of the digitalis group. There is also a bitter principle called cynotoxin, and a volatile oil.

Mode of Action: The cymarin is the primary cardioactive principle; 0.1 gm of bitter root possesses a potency of 2 U.S.P. digitalis units. Moderate doses depress the pulse and increase the contraction strength of cardiac tissue, like digitalis. It is more irritating to mucous membranes than digitalis. Perhaps this effect, as well as its marked stimulation to the vasomotor system, contributes to its diuretic action. Although it could be used as a digitalis substitute, a 1921 study found it inferior. Doses large enough to be clinically effective are too toxic to the gastrointestinal system.

Alleged Uses: Herbalists claim this to be a gallstone remedy, emetic, cathartic, and a good agent to use to "correct" bile flow. The roots and rhizomes are used to prepare an extremely bitter tonic.

Toxicity: Large doses are definitely toxic. Besides severe gastrointestinal upset, the drug will produce cardiac arrhythmias and drop blood pressure. Most poisonings are animal reports.

Comments: This is a toxic herb that should be used only under medical supervision. Bitter root is also the common name of other plants. Check genus and species names in comparing.

References: 2, 3, 9, 17, 36

Bittersweet

(*Solanum dulcamara*)
(European Bittersweet, Nightshade)

Known Principles: Bittersweets contain the glycosidal alkaloid solanine, the nonglycosidal alkaloid solanidine, the bitter dulcamarin, and two saponins, dulcamarinic and dulcamarstinic acid.

Mode of Action: The steroidal glycoalkaloids are not readily absorbed from the gastrointestinal tract but undergo hydrolysis to release free alkamines that produce the central nervous system effects. The saponins are strong irritants and produce nausea, vomiting, and a burning sensation of the mouth and throat.

Alleged Uses: Bittersweet is recommended as a "glandular" or "lymphatic" medicine by herbalists. They have also recommended it for treatment of eczema, scrofula, and syphilis, as well as a mild narcotic. Formerly it has been used for chronic rheumatism, for various skin diseases, as an aphrodisiac, and as a mild narcotic.

Toxicity: The highest concentration of the toxin is in the unripe fruit. Symptoms of burning in the throat, nausea, vomiting, decreased pulse, dizziness, increased pupil, weakness leading to muscle paralysis, headache, coma, and death may occur. As few as 2 or 3 unripe berries may produce symptoms.

Comments: This is a potentially dangerous herb that has no effect on skin disease, rheumatism, "glandular" diseases, etc. Doses high enough to give drowsiness are toxic.

References: 1, 2, 3, 17, 36

Black Alder

(Rhamnus frangula) (Frangula)
(Alder Buckthorn)

Known Principles: This plant has several glycosides in the anthraquinone class, three of which are derived from emodin. Usually black alder contains greater than 6% hydroxymethyl anthraquinone. The primary glycoside, frangulin, breaks down to the sugar rhamnose and emodin.

Mode of Action: The anthraquinones are strong, irritant cathartics. When fresh, there is also an emetic action, which dissipates if the plant is left to stand for one year.

Alleged Uses: Frangula is most often recommended as a stimulant laxative. Currently it is used more in veterinary practice than in human medicine.

Toxicity: Large amounts, or fresh black alder, will cause nausea, vomiting, severe abdominal cramps, and abdominal pain. Poisonings are rare but have occurred in Europe.

Comments: Most black alder purchased is over one year old. If purchasing any, one should be sure of this to prevent some of the emetic action. Anyone with a history of intestinal disorders should not take this without a physician's knowledge and consent.

References: 1, 2, 3, 11, 17, 23

Black Cohosh
(*Cimicifuga* spp.)

Known Principles: *Cimicifuga* contains isoferulic, palmitic, and oleic acids, as well as tannins, recemosin, 15–20% cimicifugin, and other unidentified principles. Only the cimicifugin is active.

Mode of Action: Most of its effects are likely due to its bitter nature and its astringency.

Alleged Uses: The roots and rhizomes of this plant have been used as an aid in dyspepsia.

Toxicity: Toxicity data are conflicting. Some sources (based on animal studies) suggest that the plant is nontoxic, while other sources ascribe considerable toxicity to black cohosh. In any event, toxicity may be produced with initial toxic symptoms, including nausea and vomiting. Its emetic action is not considered violent, and is probably the result of mild gastrointestinal irritation.

References: 1, 3, 5, 6, 17, 19

Black Walnut
(*Juglans nigra*)

Known Principles: Data on ingredients are sketchy and somewhat contradictory. Ingredients sometimes mentioned are nucin, juglone, and ellagic acid.

Mode of Action: Black walnut's primary action is as an astringent.

Alleged Uses: The leaves of walnuts are used to prepare a fluid extract that is used as an astringent. The leaves and bark were used against cutaneous fungal infections by the early Greeks and Romans. The nut husks contain a dark brown dye that is used in dyeing hair and clothing. The normal dose of the fluid extract is 5–10 ml.

Toxicity: Information on the toxicity of walnut leaves is not available, but their astringent nature may produce symptoms of stomach irritation. The nut kernels are edible.

References: 5, 6, 7, 16

Black Willow
(*Salix nigra*) (Pussy Willow)

Known Principles: The active principle in most willows is approximately 0.3–1% salicin. There are also tannins in the bark and the glycoside salinigrin.

Mode of Action: Salicin is a glycoside that is hydrolyzed to D-glucose and saligenin. Most likely the saligenin is then decomposed to salicylic acid in the gastrointestinal tract. The tannins are protein precipitants.

Alleged Uses: Herbalists use black willow as an astringent and antiseptic for inflamed, ulcerated surfaces. It is also a domestic remedy for rheumatoid diseases, inflamed joints, etc. Dose is 10–20 drops of the tincture.

Toxicity: There is the possibility of skin rashes; and, if taken in large amounts, salicylate poisoning is a possibility, but this would be unusual and there are no reported cases.

Comments: Tannins might be of use on open wounds, as an astringent. If salicin is converted to salicylic acid there may be some benefit to rheumatic diseases.

References: 2, 3, 17, 36

Bladderwrack
(*Fucus vesiculosus*)

Known Principles: *Fucus* contains a number of polysaccharides, including fucodin, laminarin, and alginic acid. Both iodine (0.01–0.02%) and bromine are also found.

Mode of Action: The polysaccharides are water absorbing and therefore bulk formers. A 1910 study in animals found an unidentified extract that was a stimulant to the thyroid gland.

Alleged Uses: Its primary recommended use is as a treatment for obesity. This may be due to its bulk-forming nature (full stomach) or to increased thyroid activity. Combined with other seaweeds, it has been used as a vermifuge. Other uses are similar to kelp. Dose used is 1–2 ml of the fluid extract.

Toxicity: There is no known toxicity associated with this agent.

References: 1, 9, 17

Blazing Star
(*Aletris farinosa*) (Star Grass)

Known Principles: Star grass contains the sapogenin diosgenin, a volatile oil, and an active resinous material.

Mode of Action: This herb has not been well investigated. Some sources state that any uterine action is due to the volatile oil and/or the resin material. Yet it is known that diosgenin is the substrate material used to chemically produce progesterone.

Alleged Uses: Herbalists use it for treatment of various dysmenorrhea problems and to decrease, in theory, miscarriage. The roots and rhizomes are used to expel flatulence and rheumatism, and soothe sore breasts. Normal dose is 1.3–2 gms of the dried root, or 15–40 drops of a tincture.

Toxicity: In large doses, blazing star is said to be a narcotic, emetic, and cathartic.

References: 2, 6, 36, 37, 39, 42

Blessed Thistle
(*Cnicus benedictus*)

Known Principles: Blessed thistle contains a bitter substance named cnicin and an unidentified volatile oil.

Mode of Action: The volatile oil is likely to be an irritant and the bitter principle would reflexively stimulate gastric secretions.

Alleged Uses: Its primary use is as a bitter to increase gastric secretions.

Toxicity: Large amounts act as an emetic; other toxic effects, if any, are unknown.

Comments: Useful scientific information on blessed thistle is very limited.

References: 1, 5, 9, 15

Blueberry
(*Vaccinum* spp.)
Huckleberry
(*Vaccinum myrtillus*)

Known Principles: One investigator found oleanolic and ursolic acids, beta-amyrin, myetillol, nonacosane, several fatty acids, tannins, sugar, and hydroquinone. Highbush blueberries also contain the glycoside neomyrtillin.

Mode of Action: A 1927 study showed a decrease in blood sugar after administration of an extract of blueberry leaves. The neomyrtillin has later been shown to decrease blood sugar in rabbits.

Alleged Uses: Blueberry leaf tea found its most common use against diarrhea and dysentery. It is an astringent and a diuretic approximately equivalent to uva-ursi. In Europe, it has found occasional use as an antiscorbutic.

Toxicity: No cases of toxicity were found, but data is limited. Although risk is likely low, caution should be used when using large amounts.

References: 3, 17

Blue Cohosh
(*Caulophyllum thalictroides*)

Known Principles: Besides phosphoric acid and a green-yellow dye, blue cohosh contains the saponin leontin, and the alkaloid methylcystine.

Mode of Action: *Caulophyllum* has a stimulating effect on uterine muscle but it is doubtful if this occurs in normal doses.

Alleged Uses: The roots and berries of this plant have been used as a menstrual aid and as an aid to childbirth. Heat detoxifies the berries. It has even been used as a substitute for coffee. The dose of crude plant is 0.5–1 gm.

Toxicity: Toxic symptoms include nausea, vomiting, and gastritis. Greater amounts may cause headache, thirst, dilated pupils, muscle weakness, incoordination, cardiovascular collapse, and convulsions. Since the number of berries and amount of root necessary to produce these symptoms is unclear, exposures to the uncooked plant should be treated with emesis and activated charcoal. Severely ill patients should be observed and provided with supportive care.

References: 2, 3, 4, 6, 7, 8, 17

Blue Flag
(*Iris versicolor, Iris* spp.)

Known Principles: The actual name of substances in *Iris* is confusing. It has been called iridin, irisin, and several other names. The substance seems to be a polysaccharide or oleoresin. In addition to this, there is also tannin, gum, sugar oil, a camphoraceous substance, and isophthalic acid.

Mode of Action: Iris's primary action is as a cathartic and emetic.

Alleged Uses: Eclectic physicians recommend this herb for chronic skin disorders, chronic rheumatism, and for nonmalignant enlargements and tumors. Recommended dose is 0.6–2 gms of powdered root.

Toxicity: Iris is likely to be a strong purgative, producing a burning sensation of the mouth and throat, nausea and vomiting, in addition to diarrhea. The severity is a combination of toxic effects and individual susceptibility. Skin rashes are also common.

Comments: I can see no use for Iris in treating skin diseases or "enlargements." Do not confuse this plant with sweet flat (*Acorus calamus*).

References: 1, 3, 11, 17, 36

Boneset
(*Eupatorium perfoliatum*, *E. rugosum*)
(Richweed, White Snakeroot)

Known Principles: Boneset contains the glycoside eupatorin, a volatile oil, resin, tannin, sugar, inulin, wax, and a toxic unsaturated alcohol combined with a resin acid. This alcohol, called tremetrol, may not produce symptoms when completely dry.

Mode of Action: Boneset is an emetic and an appetite stimulant. Tremetrol will decrease blood sugar but not sufficiently for toxic effects. It also appears to cause fatty degeneration of kidney and liver as well as hemorrhages in the vital organs and intestinal tract. *E. perfoliatum* probably has no virtues that cannot be attributed to its nauseating properties.

Alleged Uses: Herbalists recommend boneset against miasmatic, malarial influences, or fever. It is also used for its diaphoretic effects. Usual recommended dose is 2–4 gms of the leaves or 15–40 drops of tincture.

Toxicity: Eupatorin is a strong emetic and boneset will cause vomiting if given in large doses. *E. rugosum* is the most toxic member of the group, but is very hard to differentiate from other species. Its toxicity is reduced with drying. Symptoms of toxicity include weakness, reluctance to move, nausea, vomiting, loss of appetite, thirst, and constipation. Poisoned animals show a muscle trembling (giving the illness the name "trembles"), as well as drooling, increased respiratory rate, stiffness, coma, and death. Younger animals may be poisoned through the milk of their mothers. Humans may develop the symptoms by eating contaminated milk products, thus the illness's other name of "milk sickness." Tremetrol is excreted slowly from animals, so it may be accumulated and excreted later after the animal has been removed from the toxic plant. This plant has produced illness so devastating that during the 19th century it could cause the death of one-half of a human population through milk sickness.

References: 2, 3, 9, 11, 17, 21, 36

Buchu
(*Barosma betulina*, also called *Agathosma betulina*)

Known Principles: Buchu contains approximately 1.8% volatile oil, 30% of which is diosphenol (barosma camphor). The volatile oil has a peppermint-like odor. Buchu also contains a glycoside called diasmin, which is closely related to hesperidin, a bitter extractive, resin, 1-enthone, and mucilage.

Mode of Action: Buchu is a weak diuretic and urinary antiseptic. The volatile oil is probably antiseptic, but the quantity found in the urine is so small that antibacterial action in the bladder is unlikely. The oil is also a carminative.

Alleged Uses: Herbalists frequently recommend buchu for treatment of kidney stone, chronic prostatis, chronic inflammation of the bladder, and urethal irritation. It also finds some use as a stimulant, diuretic, and diaphoretic. Dose is 2-4 gms of the plant, or 10-20 drops of the tincture.

Toxicity: There have been no reports of toxic ingestions, but the volatile oils are irritating and may cause nausea and vomiting if taken in quantity.

Comments: This herb has all but been abandoned by the medical profession.

References: 1, 2, 3, 9, 17, 36

Buckthorn
(Rhamnus cathartica)

Known Principles: The active principles include anthraquinone glycosides equivalent to cascara. It also contains an active emetic (emodin 2%), which cascara sagrada does not.

Mode of Action: The anthraquinone glycosides are stimulant cathartics, which produce their effect by direct stimulation of the gastrointestinal tract.

Alleged Uses: The berries of this plant are pressed to release an acrid, bitter juice used in preparing the laxative, syrup of buckthorn. There are also several dyes made from this juice. The usual dose is 0.6–1.2 gms of dried berries.

Toxicity: Children exhibit symptoms of mild intoxication after consuming as few as 20 berries. Symptoms include nausea, vomiting, dizziness, and severe purging. Kidney damage may occur with large amounts. Effects may be delayed for up to six hours.

References: 1, 5, 6, 7, 8, 17

Burdock
(*Lappa* or *Arctium lappa*)

Known Principles: Several volatile oils, inulin, tannin, and a bitter glycoside called arctiin have been isolated.

Mode of Action: From the literature there do not appear to be any pharmacologically active principles in this product, although the tannins and the glycosides could have some action and should be investigated further.

Alleged Uses: The dried, first-year root or the seeds are made into an alcoholic solution to preserve the volatile oil. The tincture has been used as a remedy for "gouty" and "syphilitic" disorders and in chronic skin diseases such as psoriasis. Recommended doses are 10–15 drops of the tincture in water 3–4 times a day.

Toxicity: There seems to be little evidence that the plant has any toxic effects. However, there has been a case reported of marked anticholinergic symptoms (dilated pupils, dry mouth, hallucinations) when a commercially prepared product was used as a tea. An analysis showed marked levels of atropine. This may be due to a hereto-fore undiscovered principle in the burdock, or it may be due to a contaminated product. In any event, one should observe for these symptoms when patients ingest burdock product.

References: 10, 17, 31

Calamus Root

(*Acorus calamus*) (Sweet Root, Acore, Rat Root, Sweet Flat or Sweet Myrtle)

Known Principles: Approximately 1.5–4.5% of the plant is a bitter volatile oil. Asarone and beta-asarone make up 70–80% of this oil, the rest being eugenol, pinene, camphene, and caryophyllene.

Mode of Action: Volatile oils are generally irritating and this would give the plant some carminative properties. Its bitter taste may aid digestion by reflexly increasing acid secretion. Animal testing has demonstrated that it causes central nervous system depression. Much of this effect is thought to be due to the asarone fraction. Whether or not it has stimulant or hallucinogenic effects is questionable. If it does, it might be due to the asarone being converted in the body to the amphetamine-like hallucinogen TMA.

Alleged Uses: The root (rhizones) and overground portions are used in India in a large number of conditions including asthma, cough, flatulence, dyspepsia, convulsions, epilepsy, hysteria, insanity, and intestinal worms, or as an aphrodisiac. Doses are 1:10 infusion or 15–30 mls of tincture.

Toxicity: This herb is considered low in toxicity. Excessive amounts may cause significant drowsiness. The beta-asarone has been reported to be a hallucinogen.

References: 1, 17, 30

California Poppy
(Eschoscholtzia californica)

Known Principles: Two alkaloids, coptisine and sangui-
narine, have been isolated.

Mode of Action: Although a member of the poppy family, it
does not contain any of the morphine-codeine-like alkaloids, and the two isolated are essentially inactive.

Alleged Uses: The plant is used primarily by drug abusers for
its supposed sedative effects or "high."

References: 17, 30

Caraway
(Carum carvi)

Known Principles: Caraway seeds contain 5–7% volatile oil, a
fixed oil, proteins, and calcium oxalate. The volatile oil is
at least 50–60% the ketone carvone, and 40–50% the terpene d, l-limonene. Also present are small amounts of
carveol and dihydrocarvone.

Mode of Action: Most activity comes from the volatile oil. It is
a mucous membrane irritant and has carminative properties.

Alleged Uses: Caraway is used as an aromatic, carminative,
and flavor. As a flavoring agent, the fresh leaves are used
as a garnish and added to vegetables and other foods. It
also has flavored toothpaste. The seeds are used in bak-
ing, and the seed oil is added to ice cream, liquor, and
other foods. Medically its primary use is as a carminative

and it is often suggested as an aid for flatulent infants, for griping and cramping, and for nausea. It has even been used against scabies. Normal dose of the seeds is 1 gm; of the oil 0.1 ml.

Toxicity: There are no reported overdoses or serious harmful effects from using excessive caraway. Since it does contain significant amounts of volatile oil, the possibility of nausea, vomiting and CNS depression exists, especially in using excessive amounts of the oil itself rather than the seeds.

Comments: Medieval pharmacists called this herb *carui*; Arabians call it *karawya*.

References: 1, 2, 16, 17, 24

Cardamom Seed
(*Ellettaria cardamonum, Amonum cardamonum,* or other species)

Known Principles: Cardamom consists of 2–8% volatile oil, 3–4% starch, a nitrogenous gum, a yellow coloring matter, and a fixed oil. The volatile oil contains a terpene alcohol (borneol), and the terpenes limonene, dipentene, and terpinene.

Mode of Action: Cardamom owes its flavor and therapeutic actions to the volatile oil. The mucous membrane-irritant properties make it a useful carminative, although not as stimulating as some other volatile oils.

Alleged Uses: East Indians use cardamom as a condiment, while the Western world uses it primarily as a flavor or adjunct to other carminatives. Medicinally it is often given with other carminatives or purgatives.

Toxicity: The toxicity of cardamom is low. When used with other agents, it is seldom considered as a toxic problem. The concentration of the volatile oil is low enough so that few symptoms would be expected. The most common effects from excessive amounts of the oil are nausea, vomiting, and diarrhea.

Comments: The herb was known to the ancients and gets its name from the Greeks.

References: 1, 2, 3, 16, 17, 24

Cascara Sagrada
(Rhamnus purshiana)

Known Principles: The bark of this plant contains 6–9% anthraquinone glycosides, including cascarosides A, B, C, and D.

Mode of Action: The anthraquinone glycosides are strong stimulant cathartics. *Rhamnus* action is due primarily to increased peristalsis of the colon, although large doses may affect the upper bowel in the same manner. Cascara induces a solid or semisolid stool in about eight hours. It is not recommended for situations where the entire bowel is to be cleansed.

Alleged Uses: Cascara is used primarily as a laxative, especially with chronic constipation. Normal dose is 0.5–2 gms.

Toxicity: Excessive amounts of cascara may produce extensive diarrhea accompanied by nausea and vomiting. Severe cramping may also be present.

Comments: This herb should not be used in patients with chronic bowel disease or ulcers; it is likely to cause further injury to the bowel.

References: 17

Catalpa
(*Catalpa bignonioides*)

Known Principles: Both the bitter glycoside catalpin and catalposide have been found.

Mode of Action: Catalpin has not been well studied. Like other glycosides it has some gastrointestinal irritative effects, but support for its use in asthma has not been found.

Alleged Uses: Its primary recommendation has been for the treatment of asthma.

Toxicity: Large doses of the seeds cause nausea, vomiting, slow, weak pulse, and occasionally diarrhea. Handling the flowers has also caused some dermatitis.

References: 17

Catechu, Black
(Acacia catechu)
Catechu
(Uncaria gambier)

Known Principles: Acacia contains 25–35% catechutannic acid, catechin, quercetin, and catechu-red.

Mode of Action: These agents are astringent tannins and therefore protein precipitants.

Alleged Uses: Black catechu is recommended primarily as an astringent to decrease bleeding, decrease mucous membrane secretions, treat chronic diarrhea, and as a gargle for sore throats. Its taste is bitter and astringent. It is extracted from the wood of acacia by boiling. Normal dose is 0.3–1 gm.

Toxicity: There are no reported cases of poisonings but this is always possible with tannins. Possible symptoms range from mild to moderate bowel irritation, to kidney damage. It is probably safe to use in small amounts, but could definitely be dangerous if overused.

Comments: Catechu is a different species than black catechu, but also contains 7–33% (+)– catechin, 22–50% catechutannic acid, 34% alcohols, and 28% insoluble matter. Since its name, uses, and mode of action are approximately the same, it will not be handled separately.

References: 1, 2, 17

Catha
(Catha edulis) (Khat plant)

Known Principles: Besides several inorganic salts, tannins, and choline, catha contains several alkaloids including katine, cathine, cathinine, cathidine, and celastrin.

Mode of Action: Catha owes its usefulness to several alkaloid amines that stimulate both the brain and spinal cord. Larger doses produce paralysis through direct action upon the muscle. In 1930, cathine was found to be d-nor-pseudo ephedrine.

Alleged Uses: The green leaves are chewed or made into a tea. Their taste is sweetish and astringent, somewhat like licorice. Its primary use now is as a stimulant (like caffeine) and appetite suppressant.

Toxicity: Large doses may cause muscle paralysis and respiratory depression. Dependence has been reported. Addicts are said to experience a euphoria with loquacity, followed by apathy, depression, and anorexia. Its regular use decreases gastric secretions and may contribute to chronic gastroduodenitis and stomach disorders.

Comments: Since increased heart rate and blood pressure are possible, individuals with hypertension and heart disease should avoid this herb.

References: 1, 2, 17

Catnip
(Nepeta cataria)

Known Principles: Catnip contains a number of acids, volatile oils, and tannin. These include nepetalic acid, alpha and beta citral, limonene, dipentene, geraniol, citronella, nerol, a terpene, and acetic, butyric, and valeric acids.

Mode of Action: Catnip may be a mild central nervous system stimulant and antispasmodic. In therapeutic doses these effects are not very important since it is only a mild aromatic and slight irritant due to the volatile oil.

Alleged Uses: The leaves are infused, not boiled, or the drug is used as a snuff. It has an aromatic odor and bitter taste. Users claim it promotes sweating without increasing temperature. Its most common use is as a therapy for colic.

Toxicity: Although information on its toxicity is not available, its toxicity appears low.

Comments: Although its use in colic is not well-supported in fact, the herb appears harmless enough not to do any harm.

References: 2, 5, 9, 17

Cayenne Pepper
(Capsicum) (*Capsicum frutescens*)

Known Principles: The dried ripe fruit of this and related species contain the volatile oils capsaicine, capsacutin, and capsico. Officially, the product must have 0.5% capsaicin.

Mode of Action: The active principles are strong irritants and are used both externally as a counterirritant and internally as a gastric stimulant. When swallowed, it produces a strong sensation of heat. Although it causes intense burning if left on the skin, it seldom causes blistering. External application does not have the same effect as a rubefacient, since it affects only nerve endings, not capillaries.

Alleged Uses: Capsicum is used as an external rub or poultice and as a digestive aid or condiment. Folk medicine recommends it strongly for "purging the system of bad humors."

Toxicity: Excessive amounts cause severe irritation of mucous membranes, which may cause nausea, vomiting, and diarrhea.

Comments: This herb is usually recommended for gastrointestinal disorders. This presents a real danger if the actual medical problem is an ulcer or chronic irritation of the bowel. Bleeding and serious damage may occur in these cases.

References: 1, 17, 19

Celery Fruit
(*Apium graveolens*)

Known Principles: The seeds contain from 1.5–3% of a volatile oil consisting of approximately 60% d-limonene. The odor is due primarily to two anhydrides, sedanolid and sedanonic anhydrides. There is also some resin, a bitter extractive, and possibly high levels of nitrates in the tops.

Mode of Action: The volatile oils are mild to moderately irritating and may have some antispasmodic properties. Some studies have shown contractions of either gravid or virginal uterus.

Alleged Uses: There is a strong, but unsubstantiated belief

that celery has sedative effects. Its use for treatment of
dysmenorrhea and rheumatism is also questionable.

Comments: Large amounts of some volatile oils do produce
sedation, but this is more of a toxic than therapeutic effect.

References: 2, 3, 9, 11, 17, 24

Centuary
(*Centaurium erythraea, C. umbellatum*)
(Minor Centuary)

Known Principles: Centuary contains a colorless, crystalline,
non-nitrogenous substance called erythrocentaurin,
which is believed to be the aglycone of the glycoside
erytaurin (which is also present). More recent literature
states this compound to be a mixture of gentiopicrin,
amarogentin, and gentisin.

Mode of Action: The above agents are similar to those found
in gentian and are primarily bitter glycosides with little
pharmacologic action other than increasing gastric secretions and producing mucous membrane irritation.
(See Gentian.) The gentiopicrin has mild antimalarial action.

Alleged Uses: The summer flowers are made into an infusion
that has been used as a bitter tonic and fever reducer.
Normal dose is 1.2–2.5 gms.

Toxicity: Large amounts cause enough irritation to produce
nausea and vomiting. There are no reports of true
poisonings.

References: 1, 9, 17, 45

Chamomile
(Anthemis flores, A. nobilis)

Known Principles: The primary ingredient of chamomile appears to be a volatile oil containing tiglic acid esters. Boiling will destroy the oil. Chamomile also contains small amounts of anthemic acid (a bitter), tannic acid, resin, anthesterol, antheme, chamazulene, and apigenin (7-D-glycoside).

Mode of Action: The agent is primarily an aromatic bitter, but the volatile oil may be a mucous membrane irritant and spasmolytic. The apigenin and chamazulene are also spasmolytic agents. Chamazulene also has some anti-inflammatory and antibacterial properties. Unfortunately, both the apigenin and the chamazulene are in such small concentrations that little physiologic activity is expected.

Alleged Uses: Although all parts of this plant are utilized, the dried flower heads are most frequently used. The flowers, prepared as an infusion, liquid extract, or tea, are taken orally as an antispasmodic or digestive aid. Externally, it is applied to abscesses as a poultice.

Toxicity: Large amounts of the infusions have been reported to produce vomiting. The herb itself may cause skin rashes or serious allergic reactions in individuals known to be sensitive to ragweed pollens.

Comments: This herb should not be confused with *Matricaria chamomilla* (German chamomile).

References: 1, 3, 4, 6, 17, 48, 49, 50

Chickweed
(Stellaria media)

Known Principles: The main ingredients are potash salts and vitamin C.

Mode of Action: This plant is primarily useful only as a vitamin supplement.

Alleged Uses: The whole dried plant is prepared as an infusion. Although used internally as a demulcent, its primary use is as an ointment for external rashes and sores. The young shoots are often used in salads.

Toxicity: Human cases of temporary paralysis have been reported from large amounts of the infusion, although there is no recent evidence to indicate that chickweed presents a toxic hazard.

References: 5, 6, 12, 14

Chicory
(Cichorium intybus)

Known Principles: Chicory contains significant amounts of vitamins A and C, as well as the sugar inulin.

Mode of Action: Other than its nutrient properties, it has no medicinal action.

Alleged Uses: Chicory is commonly recommended as an edible herb. All parts are edible anytime it is seen. It is similar to dandelion in its recommended uses. Nonmedicinally, the inulin in it is used for various bacterial media.

Toxicity: Although large amounts of Vitamins A and C may

be toxic, it is very unlikely that a person would become poisoned from eating chicory.

Comments: This plant is often found as an adulterant in official dandelion preparations.

References: 2, 17, 44

Cinnamon
(*Cinnamonum camphora*)

Known Principles: Cinnamon contains gum, coloring matter, tannin, mannitol and, depending on the species, 0.5–6.0% essential oil. Cinnamaldehyde is obtained from Cassia cinnamon (a *Cinnamonum* species), or is made synthetically.

Mode of Action: The herb is a carminative and distinct astringent. It is more powerful as a local stimulant than a systemic one.

Alleged Uses: The part of the plant used is the bark. Not only is it used as a flavor but its astringency makes it useful for treatment of diarrhea and flatulence. Lately it has been mixed with marijuana and smoked by abusers.

Toxicity: Cinnamon is a strong local irritant. Skin or ocular contact will cause considerable redness and a burning sensation. Ingestions, especially of the oil, will cause nausea and vomiting. Doses of greater than 0.5 ml/kg of the oil can be dangerous enough to cause kidney damage or coma. Smaller doses produce only local effects.

References: 2, 3, 17, 22

Coconut
(Cocos nucifera)

Known Principles: Coconut contains some tannins but is mostly fixed oil. This oil (30–65% of the kernel) is made up of 50% trilaurin, 20% trimyristin, and several other glycerides including tripalmatin, tristearin, triolein, and tripalmatic acid. The last substance is what gives the oil its unpleasant odor.

Mode of Action: This agent is heavily used in manufacturing of some soaps because it does not easily precipitate in hard water or salt solutions. The oil components are used in hand cream because of their humectant and protectant properties. Portions of the plant are astringent, especially the roots. This may be the basis for which it is used as an anthelmintic.

Alleged Uses: The coconut oil is obtained by expressing the meat of the nut kernel. It is then used as an absorbable base for many pharmaceutical preparations, for scalp applications, and in both the candy and soapmaking industries. In India and Indonesia it is also used extensively to relieve toothache and as an anthelmintic.

Toxicity: There has been little in the way of toxic ingestions with this plant. The primary hazards may be in eating an excessive amount and causing some diarrhea.

Comments: Because it is not easily precipitated by salty solutions, coconut oil-based soaps are very useful as marine soaps.

References: 1, 2, 3, 16, 17

Coltsfoot
(Tussilago farfara) (Coughwort)

Known Principles: Coltsfoot contains a number of agents, including a bitter glycoside, tannin, caoutchouc, a saponin, a volatile oil, a resin, and pectin.

Mode of Action: The ingredients appear to have little activity in the concentrations used. There may be some astringency due to the tannins.

Alleged Uses: The dried leaves or flower shoots are used as a demulcent against persistent cough, like smoker's cough. Normal dose of the liquid extract is 0.6–2 mls; of the syrup, 2–8 mls.

Toxicity: There are no reported cases of coltsfoot poisoning. Since the therapeutic activity is so low, poisoning is unlikely.

References: 1, 9, 35

Comfrey
(Symphytum officinale) (Knitbone)

Known Principles: Comfrey contains mucilage, allantoin (0.6–0.8%), tannins, starch, and two alkaloids, consolidine and symphytocynglossine. Large amounts of potassium, phosphorus, and vitamins A and C have been reported.

Mode of Action: The allantoin may provide some effects in the healing of abraded skin. The tannins would be astringent and the mucilage an external demulcent.

Alleged Uses: The roots and leaves are used in poultices intended to aid in the healing of wounds and ulcers. Comfrey is also used as an internal demulcent, diuretic, and bulk laxative.

Toxicity: Toxicity is unlikely even after ingestion of moderately large quantities, but it does contain two alkaloids that have produced CNS depression in sufficient quantities. This preparation may be contraindicated in patients on dietary potassium restrictions.

References: 1, 5, 6, 17

Coneflower
(*Echinacea angustifolia, E. pallida*)

Known Principles: Coneflower contains resin, fatty acid, inulin, betaine, sucrose, and two isomeric 2-methyltetradecadienes: echinacein and echinacoside (a caffeic acid glycoside).

Mode of Action: A 1915 study found no physiologically active principles. In 1920, studies in laboratory animals could find no antibacterial benefits. There is also no proof for aphrodisiac or analgesic powers.

Alleged Uses: This is a controversial agent. Herbalists claim it is a natural antitoxin useful for both internal and external infection. The parts used most often are the roots and rhizome.

Toxicity: No reports of toxic ingestions of *Echinacea* are reported. Since it has low physiological activity, it probably is not much of a hazard.

Comments: Rudbeckia laciniata is also called coneflower and has been reported as toxic.

References: 9, 11, 17, 36

Cottonwood
(Populus deltoides, P. candicans, P. spp.)
(Balm of Gilead)

Known Principles: There is little information on cottonwood specifically, but most species contain the beta-glucoside salicin.

Mode of Action: Salicin is thought to be a salicylate precursor. Thus, sufficient quantities would be anti-inflammatory, antipyretic, and analgesic. Actual effectiveness is dependent on the quantity of plant ingested and species of cottonwood.

Alleged Uses: The bark of this tree has been used to treat everything from rheumatism and liver troubles to nasal discharge and kidney problems. Indians used it against toothache and dropsy. It is recommended for a large number of conditions that require either anti-inflammatory, antipyretic, or analgesic action.

Toxicity: The concentration of salicin is usually sufficiently low that salicylate poisoning is not a realistic concern. It is a possibility with large amounts over a prolonged period of time. Some individuals are sensitive to the pollen of these trees and develop allergies when gathering or handling certain plant parts.

References: 1, 3, 16, 39, 52

Couchgrass
(Agropyrum repens) (Dog Grass, Triticum)

Known Principles: This grass contains 2–8% sugar composed primarily of dextrose and levulose. There is some carbohydrate, inosite, gum, lactic acid, and mannite. Two glycosides have been found, one which yields vanillin on hydrolysis. If burned, the ash contains appreciable amounts of silica.

Mode of Action: Not much is known of the pharmacology involved with this plant. The sugars are said to have a diuretic effect; the glycosides have no obvious actions.

Alleged Uses: Couchgrass has been recommended as a diuretic, demulcent, nutrient, and treatment for cystitis and rheumatism. It is said to have much effect on the genitourinary organs, especially the bladder, but there are no dramatic effects noted with normal use. The recommended dose is 8–15 gms.

Toxicity: There appears to be little danger to the grass itself, but it is often contaminated with a poisonous fungus that produces ergot. Any grass containing a coating of black needs to be discarded.

Comments: This is a troublesome weed found throughout northern U.S.A.

References: 3, 6, 17, 23

Cow Parsnip
(*Heracleum lanatum*) (Hogweed, Keck)

Known Principles: This plant contains an unidentified volatile oil that is still under investigation.

Mode of Action: Specific information is lacking, but most volatile oils have varying degrees of expectorant, depressant, and spasmolytic activities.

Alleged Uses: The fruit and green parts are pulverized to make a decoction claimed to have sedative effects.

Toxicity: There have been no reports of toxicity with this plant, but not enough is yet known to truly assess its efficacy or dangers.

Comments: Some care is needed when gathering this plant since in its early stages it looks much like the poisonous hemlock.

References: 2, 45

Cranesbill
(Geranium maculatum) (Crowfoot)

Known Principles: Cranesbill contains a phlobaphene tannin (10–28%), as well as gallic acid, starch, sugar, gum, pectin, and a coloring matter.

Mode of Action: Most of cranesbill's activity appears to be due to the tannins. It is employed as an astringent and, in one 1938 study, an aqueous extract was shown to increase clotting of rabbit blood.

Alleged Uses: Naturalists recommend it as a pleasant astringent tonic for use as a mouthwash or gargle. It is used to decrease hemorrhages of the nose, mouth, stomach, or bowels. Individuals in the Appalachians used it as a treatment for dysentery and sore throat, and in poultices for external wounds.

Toxicity: Again, there is limited information concerning the toxicity of cranesbill. Since the agent contains an appreciable amount of tannin, one would suspect that severe gastritis and renal damage may occur if taken in large quantities.

Comments: Japanese beetles are attracted to this plant and die while feeding on its leaves. Therefore, it is commonly used in traps for these insects.

References: 2, 6, 17, 36, 39

Cubeb

(*Piper cubeba*) (Tailed Pepper, Java Pepper)

Known Principles: The primary ingredient (10–18%) is a volatile oil consisting of terpenes and a sesquiterpene alcohol originally called cubeb camphor. Besides this agent, 2.5–3.5% is resin, 1–3.5% cubebic acid, 0.4–3% a bitter substance called cubebin, 1% fixed oil, and 8% gum.

Mode of Action: The cubebin is virtually without physiological properties. Most of the therapeutic effects seem to come from the irritant action of cubebic acid. This substance has the ability to be absorbed and eliminated by way of the kidneys, therefore exerting an irritant action on the genitourinary tract.

Alleged Uses: The fully grown but unripe fruits are the parts used to make the preparation used medically. It is most often recommended as a diuretic and urinary antiseptic, and as an expectorant and stimulant carminative. The usual dose of the fruit is 2 gms.

Toxicity: There is little or no data on the seriousness of taking too much cubeb, but since it has an irritant, large amounts are likely to cause nausea and vomiting.

Comments: Patients with chronic or acute bowel disease should avoid this agent unless given the go-ahead by their physician. It could exacerbate any of these conditions. Arabians of the 9th and 10th centuries used it for medical purposes, but it wasn't until the 19th century that the Europeans developed an interest.

References: 1, 2, 9, 17

Damiana
(Turnera aphrodisiaca)

Known Principles: Damiana leaves contain 0.2–0.9% volatile
oil, 14% resin, approximately 3.5% tannin, 6% starch,
and a bitter substance called damianian.

Mode of Action: The volatile oil is mildly irritating, and may
induce peristalsis and gentle stimulation of the
genitourinary tract during its excretion. There appears
to be little evidence that this plant has any predictable
physiologic activity.

Alleged Uses: Damiana is prepared in both a liquid and tablet
form. Normal dose of the fluid extract is ½–1 tsp. It has a
bitter but aromatic taste and has been used as a mild
purgative, aphrodisiac, and headache remedy, and to relieve bedwetting.

Toxicity: Damiana is apparently low in toxicity, since no
documented cases of poisoning can be found.

Comments: Because of irritant action on the genitourinary
tract, patients with preexisting urinary tract disease may
have their disorders exacerbated. Caution should be
taken in these cases.

References: 2, 4, 5, 6, 30

Dandelion
(Taraxacum officinale)

Known Principles: All parts of the plant contain a bitter resin.
The concentration of the resin increases as the plant
dries. Chief constituents include teraxacerin (an acrid

resin), inulin (approximately 25%), gluten, gum, and potash. It is high in vitamins A, C and niacin. It also contains proteins, fats, and iron.

Mode of Action: The bitter principle may reflexively stimulate gastric secretions and it is a good vitamin source.

Alleged Uses: The roots and young tops are used to prepare various liquid preparations. Herbalists recommend it as a diuretic and as an aid in dyspepsia. There is no convincing reason for believing it possesses any therapeutic virtues other than its nutrient value.

Toxicity: Comparatively large doses may be ingested without toxic effects.

References: 1, 5, 6, 12, 13, 17

Elder
(*Sambucus* spp.)

Known Principles: The bark and leaves of this plant contain a purgative resin called sambucine, and a cyanogenic glycoside called sambunigrin. This glycoside yields about 0.16% hydrocyanic acid from the fresh leaves. Berries contain viburnic acid, a volatile oil, potash, lime, tyrosin, and coloring matter used as a dye. The flowers contain approximately 0.23% volatile oil, and a glycoside called rutin. The plant also contains a soft resin, albumin, wax, and tannic acid.

Mode of Action: The bark, berries, and leaves have some laxative powers. The volatile oils may have some diuretic and diaphoretic powers. The cyanogenic glycoside is, of course, toxic if taken in sufficient amounts. There is little evidence that the agents contained in this plant will cure the illnesses listed in the alleged uses section.

Alleged Uses: The berries are believed to have a cooling, refreshing effect, and serve as a laxative and diuretic. Other recommendations claim it is of use in treating headache, arthritis, gout, and phlegm of a cold. The flowers are considered a diuretic and diaphoretic, and are often used for colds, fever, and stomachaches. They are sometimes made into a poultice and applied to skin abrasions. The inner bark is a strong purgative and emetic. Indian women sometimes used it to aid the cramps of menstruation.

Toxicity: The ripe berries seem to create little toxic hazard. There have been reports of poisonings from using the stems as blowguns, and from using too much of the plant for medication. Typical poisonings include symptoms of nausea, vomiting, and general stomach distress. There is a chance of cyanide poisoning if significant amounts were to be ingested.

References: 2, 3, 6, 17, 52

Eyebright
(*Euphrasia officinalis*)

Known Principles: The precise active ingredient is unknown, but it does contain an unusual tannin, a volatile oil, and a bitter principle.

Mode of Action: Its primary action is as an astringent.

Alleged Uses: Preparations have been made from all parts of the plant except the root. The taste is saline, bitter, and slightly astringent. Eyebright is used in combination with golden seal as a lotion for eye strain and other disorders. The usual dose is 2–5 ml. of the fluid extract preparation.

Toxicity: Information on the toxicity of eyebright is not available.

Comments: Although highly recommended in many homeopathic texts, caution should be exercised in using this herb until more is known of its action.

References: 5, 6, 10

Fennel
(Foeniculum vulgare)

Known Principles: Fennel contains 2–6.5% volatile oil (which is 50–60% anethole) and 12% fixed oil.

Mode of Action: The volatile oil may produce a direct stimulant effect on the respiratory tract. It is also an aromatic stimulant and a carminative.

Alleged Uses: Fennel is used primarily as a digestive aid, cough and cold preparation, and flavoring agent. The dose of seeds is 0.3–1 g or 0.2–0.3 ml of the oil.

Toxicity: Fennel itself is not very dangerous. However, the oil extracted from it may cause skin irritation, nausea, vomiting, seizures, or pulmonary edema. Aspiration of the oil is a possibility. As little as 1–5 ml of the oil may cause symptoms.

Comments: This plant should not be confused with several other common types of fennel, including dog fennel.

References: 2, 3, 17

Fenugreek
(Trigonella foengraecum)

Known Principles: Ingredients include mucilage (28%), a strong-smelling bitter fixed oil (5%), protein, and unidentified volatile oil, the alkaloids choline and trigonelline, and a yellow dye. This product resembles cod-liver oil in that it is rich in phosphates, lecithin, organic iron, and trimethylamine.

Mode of Action: The volatile oil could be irritating to mucous membranes. Trigonelline is a metabolic breakdown product of nicotinic acid but is physiologically inert.

Alleged Uses: The seeds are used as a bulk laxative (mucilage content) and demulcent. They have a strong disagreeable odor and bitter taste.

Toxicity: No useful information on the toxicity of fenugreek could be found.

Comments: This herb is one of the prime ingredients in alleged "cure-alls" used on horses by their keepers and grooms.

References: 1, 5, 6, 17

Flaxseed
(Linum usitatissimum) (Linseed)

Known Principles: The 30–40% fixed oil, mucilage, wax, tannin, gum, and protein make up the majority of the plant, but there is also a cyanogenic glycoside called linamarin.

Mode of Action: Flax is a demulcent, an emollient, and a bulk former. It is often administered orally for its demulcent action in treatment of cough. Externally it is classified as a protective. The flax meal is used as a base for poultices, and the oil for softening the skin.

Alleged Uses: Many of its uses are as discussed in mode of action. Today its main use is as a base for preparation of poultices.

Toxicity: Linseed oil, when used as a demulcent, is considered nontoxic, and cooked flax is considered edible. The plant itself does contain, however, amounts of cyanogenic glycosides and nitrates. Overdoses have been caused by both agents. All parts contain the toxin, but immature seeds grown in warm climates have especially high concentrations. Symptoms of an overdose include an increased respiratory rate, excitement, gasping, staggering, weakness, paralysis, and convulsion.

References: 1, 2, 3, 17, 36

Fritillia
(Fritillia vericillia, F. meleagris) (Pei-Mu)

Known Principles: This herb contains several alkaloids, including fritilline, verticine, verticilline, peimine, peiminine, fritimine, and several others. The peimine and peiminine are possibly steroidal in nature.

Mode of Action: Peimine and peiminine have caused complete heart block with decreased heart rate, decreased blood pressure, and increased blood sugar when tested in animals. The fritimine has also caused hyperglycemia as well as circulatory and respiratory depression.

Alleged Uses: Fritillia is most commonly recommended as an antipyretic, expectorant, and lactagogue. The roots are the plant section utilized. There is little evidence to support these claims.

Toxicity: Some of these species have caused heart-depressant activity in Europe. Reports of poisonings are not common but there is enough activity in the alkaloids to produce serious symptoms if taken in sufficient quantities.

References: 11, 16, 17

Galanga major
(*Alpinia galanga*) (India Root, Chinese Ginger)
Galanga minor
(*A. officinarum*)

Known Principles: Galanga contains a type of oleoresin containing an oily principle called galangol, and a solid resin called kaempferid. There is also 0.5–1.5% volatile oil with small amounts of cineole and galangin.

Mode of Action: This agent is a stimulant aromatic similar to ginger. The volatile oil of *A. galanga* has antibacterial activity against a variety of Gram-positive and Gram-negative organisms.

Alleged Uses: Galanga is used as an aromatic carminative, as a treatment for impotence, sore teeth, and catarrheal afflictions, as well as a respiratory stimulant (more by reflex action than by direct stimulation). Normal dose is 1–2 gms.

Toxicity: There has been very little written about its toxicity and it must be fairly safe to use in usual doses.

Comments: This plant is related botanically and therapeutically to ginger. It has been known and utilized since the time of the ancient Greeks and Arabians.

References: 1, 2, 16, 17

Galega
(Galega officinalis) (European Goat Rue)

Known Principles: Galega contains a bitter principle, tannins, and the alkaloid galegine (which is related to synthalin).

Mode of Action: The alkaloid has been shown experimentally to produce hypoglycemia.

Alleged Uses: The plant has been tried as a treatment for diabetes, but has been replaced with more effective agents. Statements claiming it will increase breast milk have not been substantiated by animal studies. Normal recommended dose is 2–4 mls of the fluid extract.

Toxicity: There have been no reported cases of toxicity. Large amounts might produce lowered blood sugar.

Comments: This plant gives off a disagreeable odor when bruised.

References: 17

Garlic
(Allium sativum)

Known Principles: Garlic contains 0.1–0.3% of a strong-smelling volatile oil containing various allyl disulfides.

Mode of Action: Garlic's use as a larvacide and bacteriostat has been attributed to either the unstable sulfur; acrolein, or some similar unsaturated aldehyde; or a chemically undefined group of agents called phytoncides. The substance allicin, isolated from the related herb cloves, has antibacterial action equivalent to 1% of penicillin. It is active against both Gram-negative and Gram-positive organisms. Because of the irritating nature of the volatile oil, garlic also may be useful as an expectorant, diaphoretic, and diuretic.

Alleged Uses: Garlic has been used against hypertension, colic, hyperlipemia, and as an antineoplastic. There seems to be little data to substantiate most of these claims. Its use as an expectorant or externally as a rubefacient is more soundly based in fact, as are its uses as an antibacterial.

Toxicity: Fatalities have been recorded when preparations were given to children. It has also caused dermatitis. Garlic tincture has caused decreased blood pressure and leukocytosis.

References: 1, 16, 17

Gentian
(Gentiana lutea) (Other species are unofficial.)

Known Principles: Gentiopicrin, first isolated in 1862, is a glycoside that is hydrolzyed by dilute acids to release a sugar and a neutral substance called mesogentiogenin. Work in 1969 showed that mesogentiogenin was a polymer of the aglycone protogentiogenin. Other agents found in gentian include a second glycoside (gentiin), a substance related to tannins called gentiamarin, gentisin (a physiologically inert 3-monomethyl ether of 1, 3, 7, -trihydroxyflavone), gentisic acid (an organic acid), gentianose (a trisaccharide), 0.6–0.8% of the alkaloid agent gentianine, and a xanthone pigment (which could be the gentisin above). Fresh roots have about 1.5% of the gentiopicrin, the dried only about 0.1%.

Mode of Action: Usual preparations are without physiological effects except some mucous membrane irritation. It has been shown in dogs to markedly increase gastric secretions. Gentiopicrin is highly poisonous to plasmodium and therefore has been used in malaria.

Alleged Uses: The roots have been used as a bitter stomachic. They have a strong characteristic smell and a taste which is at first sweet, then profoundly bitter. Used as a stimulant to gastric secretions, it is one of the most popular of all bitters. The usual dose of 10–30 gms is usually given ½-1 hour before a meal. Its use in malaria is somewhat questionable since 4–5 pounds of the roots would be needed for a therapeutic dose.

Toxicity: In an overdose situation it acts as a local irritant and causes nausea and vomiting.

Comments: This agent has been known since the time of the Greeks and is said to have been named after a Greek king.

References: 1, 16, 17, 29

Ginger
(*Zingiber* spp.)

Known Principles: Ginger contains a number of ingredients, including cineole, citral, borneol, a yellow oil possessing phenolic properties, zingerone (a ketone related to vanillin and capsaicin), and a volatile oil. The oil consists of a sequiterpene called zingiberene, and traces of bisabolene.

Mode of Action: Ginger root is a carminative and irritant like capsicum.

Alleged Uses: Ginger is used as a carminative and as a gastrointestinal irritant for dyspepsia and griping. The root is prepared as tablets with bicarbonate, solutions, and as the pure roots. The pure root has a pleasant odor and strong pungent taste. The normal dose is 0.6–1.3 gms.

Toxicity: In general, the toxicity of this plant is low and its use in normally available (and tolerated) amounts is not expected to produce toxicity.

Comments: Patients with preexisting bowel disorders should take care if taking this herb.

References: 1, 4, 5, 6, 17

Ginseng
(Panax quinquefolium)

Known Principles: Ginseng contains a mixture of several saponin glycosides including ginenosides and panaxosides. There is also 3% volatile oil containing a camphoraceous substance, a resin, arabinose, mucilage, and starch.

Mode of Action: Ginseng can best be termed an "adaptogen." It allows the body to adapt to certain biological stresses. Panaxin is a stimulant for midbrain, heart, and blood vessels. Panax acid is a stimulant to the heart and to the general metabolism. Panaquilin stimulates internal secretions, and panacen and sapogenin are volatile oils that stimulate the central nervous system. Ginsenin is an agent that decreases blood sugar. Ginseng in general has a stimulant effect on the adrenal cortex. Corticosteroid content in the urine is increased by more than 60% and the eosinophil cell count is decreased after administration of ginseng. There have been experiments that conclude that ginseng increases both mental and physical efficiency. During stress the amount of vitamin C is decreased in the adrenals. When ginseng is administered, the time of decreased vitamin C concentration is shortened and there is a more rapid return to a normal level. This may contribute to ginseng's property as a adaptogen. Ginseng also stimulates an aerobic and anaerobic glycolysis in the liver and kidneys with no significant increase in oxygen consumption. Ginseng is also a histamine liberator, probably attributable to the saponin content of the extracts. There is also direct effect on muscles since ginseng affects expenditure of energy stored in muscle ATP. This allows for better skeletal muscle tonus and weight gain. Therefore, ginseng has been called a "biocatalyzer."

Alleged Uses: Ginseng has been recommended for almost everything. It is a favorite Chinese remedy, especially for impotence. Ginseng has also been recommended for the treatment of anemia, atherosclerosis, depression, diabetes, edema, hypertension, stress, and ulcers. The normal dose administered is 1–4 gms.

Toxicity: Poisoning by ginseng is not common. Cases of overdose have not been reported. There are, however, a number of glycosides in ginseng. Therefore, caution should be taken in using excessive amounts of this herb.

Comments: The ginseng plant is native to Georgia and is currently under consideration for legislative protection in that state.

References: 1, 2, 3, 16, 23

Golden Seal
(*Hydrastis* spp.)

Known Principles: The rhizome contains 1–3% hydrastine (an alkaloid), 3–4% berberine, and traces of candine, resin, albumin, starch, fats, sugar, lignin, and a volatile oil. The most active constituent is the hydrastine, while berberine is practically inert.

Mode of Action: The mechanism of action for its use in decreasing uterine bleeding is unknown, but this action is much inferior to that of ergot. Hydrastine has little effect on the CNS in subtoxic doses; however, in toxic doses it can produce convulsions. Parenteral administration of the fluid extract produces little effect in low doses unless given I.V., when hypotension results. This hypotension is probably due to a direct myocardial depressant effect. It also has a depressant effect on intestinal smooth muscle.

Alleged Uses: The dried rhizome is the portion of the plant used medicinally although all parts contain the active ingredients. Its taste is very bitter and it has been used as a bitter for dyspepsia as well as an aid to stop postpartum bleeding. It is usually taken in doses of 1–2 gms (of the rhizome).

Toxicity: Large amounts are poisonous, producing irritation of the mouth and throat, nausea, vomiting, diarrhea, and paresthesia. Fatalities result from central nervous system stimulation, paralysis, and respiratory failure. The paralysis comes from a depressant effect on the spinal cord and peripheral nerves. Its effects on circulation vary; there is no consistent information. Its effects in decreasing uterine hemorrhage may be related to increased stimulation of the uterine muscle, resulting in a decreased bleeding.

Comments: This herb is potentially dangerous and should not be used without proper medical consultation.

References: 1, 3, 4, 5, 6

Gotu Cola
(*Cola nitida*) (Kola)

Known Principles: Kola contains up to 3.5% caffeine and 1% theobromine, as well as some catechol and epicatechol. In the fresh nuts the caffeine is combined with a tannin called kolacatechin.

Mode of Action: Both of the above xanthines are noted for central nervous system stimulation and diuretic actions. The fresh nuts are also astringent, possibly related to either the tannin or catechol.

Alleged Uses: The herb is used to decrease fatigue and increase diuresis, and the seed kernels are used as a "chewing stimulant." Another major use is as a flavoring agent. The normal dose is about 4 gms (teaspoon).

Toxicity: Kola is generally considered to be low in toxicity, but excessive use could cause nervousness, insomnia, or increased heart rate, or aggravate peptic ulcer.

Comments: There are several species called gotu cola. *C. nitida* contains caffeine; others may not. For example, another plant commonly called Gotu Kola is *Hydrocotyle asiatica major*, which is not related to the kola group, and does not contain caffeine.

References: 17, 24, 29, 30

Grape Hyacinth
(Muscari racemonsum, M. comosum)

Known Principles: This plant is said to contain cosmisic acid.

Mode of Action: Cosmisic acid has saponinlike action; therefore, strong gastrointestinal irritation could be expected.

Alleged Uses: Grape hyacinth is occasionally recommended for diuresis and as a stimulant.

Toxicity: The bulb is reportedly toxic. Symptoms would be nausea, vomiting, and profuse diarrhea.

Comments: There is little evidence that this has a useful therapeutic effect that warrants exposing oneself to the toxic effects.

References: 2, 6

Grindelia
(Grindelia camporum, G. humilus, G. squarrosa)
(Gumweed)

Known Principles: Gumweed's activity is most likely related to an amorphorus balsamic resin that constitutes 16–21% of the herb. Traces of a bright yellow volatile oil, a hydric alcohol called grindelol, tannins, and robustic acid have also been found. Some claim to have found alkaloids and saponins, but these agents have not been substantiated.

Mode of Action: Grindelia appears to have only weak physiologic powers. Large doses produced drowsiness, mydriasis, decreased heart rate, and increased blood pressure in animals. It acts primarily on nerves and muscles. This action may be correlated with the fact that the

Grindelia species can accumulate selenium. Animal studies showed first a stimulating, then a depressant action on the heart. It also appears to be a stimulant expectorant.

Alleged Uses: Primarily, Grindelia is used as an expectorant and mild sedative. Some claim it has spasmolytic actions as well and therefore, it is commonly used to treat asthma and bronchitis. It reportedly has a bad taste. This plant has been applied locally to burns and vaginitis and used in various poultices.

Toxicity: Toxic ingestions are not common, but the active resins are excreted renally; therefore, large doses may produce renal irritation.

References: 1, 5, 6, 11, 17

Guaiac
(*Guaiacum officinale* or *G. sanctum*)

Known Principles: Approximately 18–25% of guaiac is composed of resin, of which 70% is guaiaconic acid. There is also 10% guaiaretic acid, 15% vanillin, a saponin, and a coloring agent known as guaiac yellow.

Mode of Action: Most of guaiac's effects are caused by the resin. They have a local irritant effect on the gastrointestinal tract and stimulate sweating. It is doubtful that it has much therapeutic effect other than as a nauseant.

Alleged Uses: Guaiac was previously classified as an "alternative" drug, and used for all kinds of chronic, difficult to cure diseases such as syphilis, chronic rheumatism, and scrofula. Today it is used primarily as a laxative and diuretic and is no longer recommended for skin diseases or rheumatism. The resin, which is obtained by boiling wood chips, is usually taken in doses of 0.3–2 gms. The most common use for guaiac currently is as a test for oxidizing enzymes. This principle is applied for detection of occult blood. The reaction is blood plus hydrogen peroxide plus guaiac equals a blue color.

Toxicity: Poisonings are not a common problem, but since it is a gastrointestinal irritant, large amounts will cause nausea and vomiting. This has occasionally been seen even with therapeutic doses.

References: 1, 2, 8, 9, 16, 17

Hawthorn
(*Crataegus* spp.)

Known Principles: Hawthorn contains cratagolic acid, a mixture of saponins, triterpene acids (e.g., oleanolic, ursolic, crataegolic), purines, and anthocyanin-type pigments. English hawthorn is also reported to contain some flavonoid glycosides.

Mode of Action: Graham (1940) found tincture of *Crataegus* orally had very little effect on experimental animals, but when given intravenously, it depressed both respiration and heart rate. The animals had an initial decrease in blood pressure followed by cardiac arrhythmias and heart failure. It also relaxed uterine and intestinal smooth muscle but constricted both the bronchi and the coronary artery. In 1951 Ullsperger isolated a yellow substance from English hawthorn that dilated coronary blood vessels. This was later tried on 100 patients with beneficial results, either subjectively or by decreasing their dose of digitalis.

Alleged Uses: It is recommended primarily for decreasing high blood pressure.

Toxicity: There have been no toxic ingestions reported, but the possibility for adverse cardiac effects is certainly present.

Comments: Although this agent may appear to have some beneficial cardiac effects, it has been supplanted by other agents with higher potency and better therapeutic effects.

References: 1, 17

Heliotrope
(Heliotropium europaem)

Known Principles: This herb contains the pyrrolizidine alkaloids heliotrine and lassiocarpine.

Mode of Action: After ingestion the liver cells increase in size, have an increased death rate, and lose their regenerative powers. Liver dissection shows a small amount of fibrosis.

Alleged Uses: This herb is not commonly recommended as a medication, but people become exposed to it because it becomes mixed in home-grown-and-gathered grains. It is also sometimes mistaken for valerian because of valerian's common name of garden heliotrope.

Toxicity: This plant is a slow-acting liver toxin responsible for extensive livestock damage. Younger animals are more susceptible than older ones.

Comments: Heliotrope is a common weed.

References: 11, 16, 21

Hellebore

(Veratrum viride)

(American Hellebore, Green Hellebore)

Known Principles: Hellebore contains a large number of steroidal glycoalkaloids. These include jervine, pseudojervine, rubijervine, cevadine, germitrine, germidine, vertralbine, veratroidine, to name just a few. Most important therapeutically are germidine and germitrine.

Mode of Action: The pharmacologic effects of hellebore are complex. Briefly stated, the veratrum alkaloids produce a reflex depression of blood pressure and heart rate and have some sedative properties. Small doses seem to decrease the blood pressure with little effect on the respiratory rate or cardiac rate. The alkaloids are absorbed from the gastrointestinal tract, although somewhat variably. There is little information regarding the distribution of the active constituents in the body or the excretion of these alkaloids. Active preparations of veratrum alkaloids cause a decrease in both systolic and diastolic peripheral blood flow. The fall in blood pressure results from reflex vasoconstrictor mechanism, which is the sympathetic portion of the autonomic nervous system. There is no direct dilating action on the peripheral vessels and no ganglionic blocking or adrenergic blocking action. The hypotensive action can be prevented or corrected by sypathomimetic amines such as ephedrine. The hypotensive action is proportional to the dose administered and is independent of the change in heart rate.

With therapeutic doses, orthostatic hypotension is infrequent. Bradycardia is also of reflex origin.

The pulse rate decreases to about 60/minute under the influence of the drug, but epinephrine and similar drugs will still increase the rate as usual. Cardiac output is unchanged unless an excessive dose causes vascular collapse. Peripheral blood flow is increased in the extremities, kidney, and liver, but does not change in sympathectomized extremities. In usual doses, there is no significant effect on renal function. Respiration is affected only by doses larger than those required to affect the cardiovascular system and will produce respiratory failure.

Alleged Uses: Hellebore has been used by both herbalists and traditional physicians in the treatment of hypertension especially associated with toxemia of pregnancy. It has also been used as a circulatory depressant, stomachic, emetic, or parasitic agent. The normal dose is around 100 mg of the plant. It may also be administered as 1:10 tincture. The dose of this is 0.3–2 mls. The unstandardized official preparation, which is of the dried rhizomes and roots, often is very weak and of even questionable action. On oral administration, the effect of an antihypertensive dose and a toxic dose are so close together as to make effective use of veratrum preparations impractical in many patients because of changing individual sensitivity to the drug. Parenterally, the alkaloidal preparations are valuable and safe if used with caution.

Toxicity: All parts of the plant are toxic, especially the roots. The danger appears to be greatest in early spring growth. Symptoms of poisoning include a burning sensation of the mouth, drooling, nausea, vomiting, diarrhea, stomach pain, headache, prostration, decreased heart rate, and hypotension. Poisoning rarely is fatal because of rapid vomiting and poor absorption.

References: 1, 3, 5, 7, 8, 9, 11, 17

Helonias
(*Chamaelirium luteum*)
(False Unicorn Root, Fairy Wand)

Known Principles: This herb is said to contain 9.5% of the saponin glycoside chamaelirin.

Mode of Action: The herb is an emetic, diuretic, and potential vermifuge, as well as a strong local irritant. It is doubtful that it has any value in the treatment of uterine disorders.

Alleged Uses: The roots and rhizomes are used to prepare bitter, astringent teas and tinctures, recommended for prevention of miscarriages, problems of menopause, increasing appetite, and reducing colic.

Toxicity: Chamaelirin is one of the least toxic of the saponins. Large doses will produce nausea and catharsis.

Comments: The bitter taste may increase appetite reflexively and the local irritant effect may serve as an expectorant.

References: 2, 6, 17, 36, 39

Henbane
(*Hyoscyamus niger*) (Hyoscyamus)

Known Principles: Officially henbane must contain greater than 0.04% alkaloid. Usually it contains from 0.05–0.15% of the two alkaloids hyoscyamine and scopolamine. The percentage varies greatly with the age of the plant. The young plant contains larger amounts of scopolamine, older plants have more hyoscyamine. A mature plant contains ¾ hyoscyamine.

Mode of Action: Similar to belladonna in its action, it is a parasympatholytic. It has little effect on blood vessels but in larger amounts will increase heart rate, cause dilated pupils, dryness of the mouth, urinary retention, and hallucinations, and reduce intestinal peristalsis.

Alleged Uses: Although listed in most herbals as a poison, it is used in somewhat smaller doses for its antispasmodic action with whooping cough and asthma. It has also been used as a mouthwash for toothache, a solution for earache, to induce sleep, or decrease pain.

Toxicity: This substance is poisonous to children and animals. Symptoms include dilated pupils, increased heart rate, delirium, and most of the symptoms listed above. As little as 1–2 mg can cause significant symptoms. This is as little as 20 gms of the raw plant.

Comments: Has a sticky stem and nauseating odor. This plant was thought by the ancients to have magical powers.

References: 1, 2, 6, 8, 11, 17, 47

Hop
(*Humulus lupulus*)

Known Principles: Ingredients include approximately 0–1% humulene (a sesquiterpen volatile oil), lupulinic acid, and lupulon (two bitter principles).

Mode of Action: Hops are an aromatic bitter. Both of the bitters the plant contains have antiseptic properties. The volatile oil seems to be inert. Hops are reported to have a central nervous system depressant activity on frogs, birds, and mice, but human data are unavailable.

Alleged Uses: The fruit of this plant is concentrated in the form of an infusion or tincture, then administered as a tonic for dyspepsia and diuresis. If the fruit is not fresh, valerianic acid is formed, which imparts an unpleasant odor to preparations made with this product.

Toxicity: There is little data on the toxicity of hops. They appear to have a low toxic potential.

Comments: Do not confuse this herb with wild hops (*Bryonia* spp.), which is toxic. Hops are used extensively in the brewing industry.

References: 3, 4, 5, 6, 16, 17

Horehound
(*Marrubium vulgare*)

Known Principles: Horehound contains a volatile oil, a resin, a tannin, and a very bitter principle called marrubiin (a hydroxyditerpene lactone).

Mode of Action: The volatile oil is a carminative and expectorant, while the bitter will give reflex gastric action.

Alleged Uses: Horehound has long been a domestic remedy for coughs and colds, as an expectorant and aromatic stimulant, a diaphoretic, and an irritant. The leaves and flowers are used to make a tincture. Horehound was once considered an antimagic herb.

Toxicity: There have been no reports of toxic ingestions or misuses. Large amounts do cause diarrhea and nausea, so some care should be taken in the amount one uses.

References: 6, 17, 36, 37, 39

Horse Chestnut
(Aesculus hippocastanum)

Known Principles: The bark of horse chestnut contains the toxic coumarin glycoside aesculin. It also has the hemolytic saponin escin and the glycosides argyroscin and capsuloescinic acid. The latter two do not seem to be of any medical importance. The seeds have 49% starch and approximately 4% oil.

Mode of Action: Injection of a horse chestnut extract caused an increase in capillary and red cell resistance and an increase in plasma antithrombin activity, causing increased bleeding times. Besides their hemolytic effect, horse chestnuts are mucous membrane irritants and will cause nausea and vomiting.

Alleged Uses: At one time this agent was tried as an anticoagulant. It has been replaced by more reliable, less toxic agents. Since the aesculin absorbs ultraviolet light, a 4% solution has been used in solutions as a sunscreen.

Toxicity: Typical overdoses cause nausea, vomiting, inflamed membranes, increased temperature, incoordination and hemolysis. Even a few nuts can be serious.

Comments: There is some evidence that nuts or plant parts in a small pond will stupefy the fish.

References: 2, 3, 11, 17, 21, 26

Horsemint
(Monarda punctata and other species)

Known Principles: Horsemint's primary principle is known as monarda oil. It is composed of 60% thymol and smaller amounts of cyemene, d-limonene, carvacrol, linalool, and hydrothymoquinone.

Mode of Action: Thymol is a powerful disinfecting agent, even more so than phenol. It is irritating to the tissues and is bacteriocidal. Its ability to kill microorganisms is significantly reduced by the presence of proteins. Almost 50% of this oil is excreted in the urine, making it slightly useful as a urinary antiseptic.

Alleged Uses: The primary uses have been as both an external and internal fungicide, anthelmintic, and bacteriocide. The mint has an aromatic odor and a warm, bitter taste. The tea is used as a carminative for colic, flatulence, and sick stomach. Winnebago and Dakota Indians used an infusion as a heart stimulant.

Toxicity: There have been no reports of toxic ingestions. Rashes are common with external use. The thymol is slightly more toxic than phenol, which is considered toxic in doses of 1–5 gms. A significant amount of plant material would be needed to obtain this much oil.

References: 1, 2, 3, 16, 17, 34

Horseradish

(*Armoraciae radix*, also called *Cochlearia armoracia*)

Known Principles: This herb contains the glycoside sinigrin, which when combined with water and the enzyme myrosin releases the volatile oil containing allyl isothiocyanate.

Mode of Action: The external application will induce inflammation and vesiculation. Internally it is an intense irritant. Vapors of crushed horseradish seem to have an inhibitory effect on microorganisms.

Alleged Uses: Horseradish is used as a stimulant to the digestive system much like mustard, but it is less potent.

Toxicity: Eating large amounts of the raw root has caused bloody vomiting and diarrhea.

References: 3, 17

Horsetails
(Equisetum spp.) (Shave Grass, Bottle Brush)

Known Principles: Horsetails contain appreciable amounts of silica, aconitic acid, equisitine, starch, several fatty acids, and even some nicotine.

Mode of Action: This plant is strongly astringent and most activities are a result of this action.

Alleged Uses: A fluid extract is prepared from the barren stems of this plant and is used as both an external and internal astringent for treatment of skin sores, diarrhea, dyspepsia, and diuresis.

Toxicity: This plant is toxic in excesses. Children have been poisoned by using the stems as blow guns or whistles. Symptoms in animals include muscle weakness, ataxia, weight loss, abnormal pulse rate, cold extremities, and fever. Most of these symptoms were reported after chronic ingestions by the animals.

Comments: Patients with hypertensive disease and/or other cardiovascular problems should not consider using this agent.

References: 3, 5, 6, 16, 22

Houseleek

(Sempervivum tectorum, Sempervivum spp.)
(Jupiter's Eye, Thor's Beard)

Known Principles: Houseleek contains malic acid and a limelike substance.

Mode of Action: Malic acid should be slightly astringent as are many other organic acids. The mode of action of the limelike substance is unknown.

Alleged Uses: The leaves are made into juice, which is used as an astringent and diuretic. These plants are most commonly used in a poultice for treatment of insect stings, burns, bruises, and various skin diseases.

Toxicity: In large doses houseleeks are emetics and purgatives, but there is little evidence that the plant is a serious toxic hazard.

References: 3, 4, 5, 6

Hydrangea

(Hydrangea paniculata) (Seven-Barks)

Known Principles: Hydrangeas contain two resins, a sulfur-containing volatile oil, a saponin, and the cyanogenic glycoside hydrangin. The leaves and buds have hydrangin; the roots are the part usually made into medicine.

Mode of Action: The volatile oil is likely to be carminative and slightly astringent. The activity of the resins and saponins has not been fully explored.

Alleged Uses: Once this plant was thought to be a stimulant and was used to reduce calculus of the bladder and cystitis. It is no longer recommended for these uses. American pioneers tried it to treat dyspepsia. Currently it is being used as a marijuana substitute because of its supposed stimulant activity.

Toxicity: Excessive amounts cause dizziness, an oppressed feeling of the chest, and nausea and vomiting. Livestock poisoning symptoms have not been consistent with cyanide poisoning; therefore, there is most likely activity from some other compound as well. Under normal conditions, hydrangeas are minimally or nontoxic.

References: 3, 11, 16, 17, 22

Indian Nettle
(*Acalypha indica, A. virginica*)
(Kuppi, Mercury Weed)

Known Principles: The alkaloid acalyphine is found throughout the plant, as is a cyanogenic glycoside that is actively poisonous. Resin, volatile oil, inositol methyl ether, and triacetomamine are also found.

Mode of Action: The plant is known to have emetic and expectorant activities similar to those of ipecac. Whether this is due to the alkaloid or to the volatile oil has not been determined.

Alleged Uses: The plant is used both dried and fresh as an expectorant and laxative. Indians used the fresh leaves in a poultice for ulcers, as a vermifuge, and in a suppository for constipated children. Occasionally it has been applied as a mouthwash for sore gums. The normal dose of the liquid extract is 0.3–2 mls.

Toxicity: There have been no reports of toxic ingestions with this plant.

References: 3, 9, 16, 17

Indigo, Wild
(*Baptisia tinctoria*)

Known Principles: *Baptisia* has several phenolic glycosides including baptisin, baptisine, and bapitoxine. Bapitoxine is identical to cytisine. Several quinolizidine alkaloids have also been found. The blue dye it contains is said to be inferior to regular indigo.

Mode of Action: Most of the glycosides have minimal activity. Cystisine is a strong emetic and cathartic but this is likely to be its only activity.

Alleged Uses: Herbalists have recommended this for a number of septic conditions, including typhoid fever and amoebic dysentery. The dried roots are used both internally and externally, but there is little evidence that it is a germicide. Normal dose of tincture is 2–20 drops.

Toxicity: Overdoses of this plant cause severe diarrhea, vomiting, and loss of appetite. It has caused poisonings in both humans and animals.

References: 2, 3, 11, 17, 36

Irish Moss
(*Chondrus crispus, Gigartina mamillosa*)

Known Principles: Almost 55–80% of Irish Moss is a pectin-like substance known as carrageenan, a mucilaginous principle. The product also contains approximately 10% protein and a number of minerals such as calcium, sodium, potassium, magnesium, chlorine, iodine, and bromine. The carrageenan is chemically similar to, yet different from, agar.

Mode of Action: The protectant and demulcent uses of Irish moss are attributed to the carrageenan. An investigator in 1937 showed a nitrogenous, polysaccharide, sulfuric ester related to heparin. It also has an anticoagulant effect. In 1939 a patent was granted for this substance.

Alleged Uses: The main use of Irish moss is as a bulk former, protector, and dumulcent. It is used in this manner in the OTC drug Kondremul. It is also said to have anticoagulant powers equal to that of heparin and it claims use as a demulcent in the treatment of coughs or diarrhea. Besides its medical uses, it is used as a soothing hand lotion, as a substitute for gelatin in jellies, and even as a suspending agent in toothpaste. The usual dose as a demulcent is about 15 gms.

Toxicity: There does not appear to be any serious toxicity from Irish moss. Caution may be taken for those individuals with bowel obstruction.

Comments: There exists a possible interaction of Irish Moss and any anticoagulant. Therefore, individuals on anticoagulant therapy should take special care if using Irish moss.

References: 1, 2, 16, 29, 34

Jalap Root
(Exagonium purga) (Conqueror Root, High John Root, Ipomea, Turpeth)

Known Principles: Jalap root contains 8–12% glycosidal resin called both jalapin or convolvulin. It has a molecular weight near 31,018 and is most likely composed of glycosides and methy-pentosides of jalapinolic acid. A volatile oil, a starch, a gum, and a sugar are also found in the herb.

Mode of Action: The resin is a moderately strong purgative. It has an irritant action on the intestinal tract and produces profuse, watery diarrhea. It is said to cause purging even if applied to an open wound.

Alleged Uses: Jalap is primarily recommended as a cathartic. The dose of the powder is 1 gm; the range is 0.3–1.2 gms.

Toxicity: Overdoses of this drug may cause dangerous hypercatharsis with fluid and electrolyte loss.

Comments: The name of this plant has changed a number of times over the years.

References: 1, 2, 6, 17, 21

Jamaican Dogwood
(Piscidia erythrina) (Fish-Poison Tree)

Known Principles: Jamaican dogwood contains the substance piscidin, which is a mixture of two glycosides related to rotenone and is poisonous to fish.

Mode of Action: Experiments on animals have shown this herb will poison fish and make dogs react as if they had taken cannabis. This latter action is weak, however, being only 1/17 as strong as cannabis itself. Jamaican dogwood has also shown some anodyne properties and has shown a potent uterine depressant action in laboratory animals.

Alleged Uses: Naturalists claim Jamaican dogwood is a narcotic, useful in treating various nervous conditions. It has also been recommended for dysmenorrhea and for hysteria. The bark is the portion used, and it is said to produce a burning sensation in the mouth and throat when ingested.

Toxicity: Animal studies indicate this substance has no toxicity (except for fish). It appears to be mildly narcotic, but not really dangerous.

Comments: Bark has been used for catching fish in some primitive countries. The pulverized bark is put in a basket that is dragged through a stream until fish are stupefied. The bark is said to have an odor like opium.

References: 3, 17, 36

Jequirity Bean
(Abrus precatorius) (Crab's Eyes, Indian Licorice, Rosary Pea)

Known Principles: Jequirity contains abric acid, the amino acid abrive, N-methyltrytophan, the lipolytic enzyme hemoglutin, a glycoside, and the thermolabile toxalbumin abrin. The roots, stems, and leaves have traces of glycyrrhizin; thus the name Indian licorice.

Mode of Action: Abrin is an extremely toxic agglutinating phytotoxin that will cause cell destruction in the same manner as many bacterial toxins. When placed in the eye it produces a severe reaction that increases circulation, therefore promoting absorption of inflammatory exudates. If inappropriately used, this procedure can do more harm than good and has been responsible for causing blindness.

Alleged Uses: Abrin's primary use in the past was as a 1/500,000 solution that was instilled into the eyes for various types of chronic eye disorders. It is no longer used therapeutically but still comes to our attention due to accidental or intentional poisonings.

Toxicity: Jequirity beans are most toxic when chewed. Swallowing them whole greatly reduces the danger because the toxalbumin is not absorbed well through the hard seed coat. If a bean is chewed, one experiences a caustic burning of the mouth, resulting in oral burns, severe nausea, vomiting, diarrhea, increased heart rate, blood in the urine, red cell destruction, convulsions and death. Symptoms might not appear for several hours or even days after ingestion because of the erratic absorption of the material inside the seed coat. As little as one seed has been reported to cause serious symptoms. The estimated lethal dose of abrin is 0.1 mg per kg of body weight of the victim.

Comments: This is a common weed in Florida and Central and South America. Although seldom used medically today, the seeds are so colorful that they are commonly strung as a necklace and given to children. The risks in doing this are obvious.

References: 1, 2, 3, 6, 8, 16, 17

Jersey Tea
(*Ceanothus americanus*) (Red Root)

Known Principles: Jersey tea contains 10% tannin, resin, oil, ceanothic acid, and 3 alkaloids. The blood coagulant substance appears to be a mixture of succinic, oxalic, malonic, orthophosphoric, and pyrophosphoric acids.

Mode of Action: The root, which gives a red color in water, is an astringent. Although once used to treat syphilis, there is no reason to believe it has any value. There has been a commercial product prepared and recommended for use to increase coagulability of blood. An extract of this plant used in a 1922 study demonstrated a decrease in blood pressure and in coagulation. Other studies have shown similar results.

Alleged Uses: Red root has often been recommended as a "spleen" remedy, and as an astringent, expectorant, sedative, antispasmodic, and antisyphilitic. It is especially recommended for despondency and melancholy. Dose of tincture is 10–20 drops.

Toxicity: There have not been many reports of toxic ingestions, but chronic users may wish to have their coagulation time checked.

Comments: There is a commercial product called Ceanothyn that is used for clotting purposes.

References: 2, 17, 36, 39

Jimson Weed

(*Datura stramonium*)

(Sacred Datura, Thorn Apple)

Known Principles: Jimson weed contains atropine, hyoscyamine and a trace of scopolamine. Total alkaloid content is approximately 0.25–0.7%.

Mode of Action: This is an anticholinergic agent; effects are
related primarily to antagonism of acetylcholine com-
petitively at the neuroreceptor site. Heart, brain, smooth
muscle, and most exocrine glands are affected by these
agents. *Datura* has found some use in the treatment of
asthma since atropine paralyzes the vagus nerve ending
in the pulmonary branch, thus relieving bronchospasms.

Alleged Uses: Historically, Jimson Weed has been used in the
treatment of various respiratory diseases, especially
asthma, and for several nonspecific types of dyspepsia.
More recently it has been smoked or brewed as a tea for
its hallucinogenic effect.

Toxicity: Four to five gms of crude leaf (1–2 tsp.) approaches
the fatal dose for a child. Although all parts contain the
toxic agent, the highest concentration is in the seeds.
Symptoms of dry mouth, dilated pupils, flushing, increased temperature, headache, increased heart rate, increased blood pressure, heart beat abnormalities, convulsions, hallucinations, and coma are possible. Skin contact
may produce skin rashes. Ingestions of this plant have
been fatal.

References: 2, 3, 17, 22

Juniper
(Juniperus communis or *J. depressa)*

Known Principles: The dried ripe fruit contains 0.5–2% volatile oil and about 10% resin, 33% sugar, tannin, and a flavone glycoside. Not less than 0.5 ml of juniper oil should be obtained from each 100 gms of the berries. The highest concentration of the volatile oil is in the full-grown, but unripe berries. The riper the berries, the more of the volatile oil has been converted to the resin form. The volatile oil has been called oil of sabinal. The oil is obtained by steam distillation and contains 50% alcohols, primarily 1-terpinen-4-ol, alpha-pinene, camphene, and cadinene.

Mode of Action: Whatever supposedly therapeutic value juniper has is attributed to the volatile oil. The local irritant effect of the volatile oil is capable of producing injurious effects to the kidney, especially if that organ is already inflamed.

Alleged Uses: Used for its stimulant effect in chronic disorders of the genitourinary tract, juniper oil was one of the ingredients in many of the "patent" medicines recommended for diuretic effects. Other uses include: carminative for colic and flatulence, an abortifacient, and as a flavoring in gin and other alcoholic beverages. Normal recommended dose is 0.06–0.3 mls of the oil.

Toxicity: A single large dose gives only catharsis, but smaller repeated doses may produce personality changes, renal damage, or convulsions.

Comments: Older copies of the United States Dispensatory had definite standards set up to control this agent.

References: 1, 17, 29

Kava-Kava
(*Piper methysticum*)

Known Principles: There are two yellow pigments called flavokawin A and flavokawin, as well as several alkaloids of the alpha-pyrone type. These include methysticin, dihydromethysticin, kawain, dihydrokawin and demethoxyyangonin.

Mode of Action: The primary effect of the alkaloids is to produce drowsiness. The pigments are also known to produce skin pigmentation and lesions, but the mechanism is unknown.

Alleged Uses: This herb has generally been recommended as a sedative against anxiety and fatigue. It is also recommended as a diuretic and a genitourinary antiseptic, even for the treatment of gonorrhea.

Toxicity: Acute doses appear to give only mild sedation, but chronic low-dose administration has caused skin coloring and skin lesions.

References: 1, 30

Kelp
(May be members of several genera, such as *Laminaria*, *Fucus*, or *Sargassum*)

Known Principles: Kelp has been known as a reliable source of both iodine and bromine for some time. It is also a rich source of alginic acid.

Mode of Action: Alginates (salt forms of alginic acid) have greater water-absorbing and retaining properties than methyl cellulose, and they do not swell up in an acid environment. This makes them especially useful as a bulk laxative. The acid-neutralizing and buffering actions along with hemostatic properties make it useful for treatment of ulcers.

Alleged Uses: Alginates have found several uses in both medicine and industry. Various salts forms are used for such things as thickening and stabilizing agents, treatment of gastric ulcers, and stool softeners.

Toxicity: Kelp appears to be almost nontoxic. Large amounts could produce some iodine toxicity but this is unlikely.

References: 2, 3, 17

Knot Weed
(*Polygonum aviculare*) (Pigweed)

Known Principles: A 1928 study found 0.2–0.8% emodin, the glycoside quercetin 3-arabinoside, and avicularin.

Mode of Action: Quercetin is a bioflavonoid glycoside. Members of this group reduce capillary permeability induced by histamine or by tissue injury, decrease capillary fragility (by increasing the tensile strength of capillary walls), and retard the destruction of epinephrine by body tissue. Although members of this group have sometimes been called vitamin P, there is no evidence they have any true vitamin function. Their therapeutic value is questionable. The emodin would serve as a cathartic, however, and its effectiveness is related to amounts ingested.

Alleged Uses: Herbalists call this a "gravel" remedy for removal of kidney and bladder stones. The recommended dose is 10–20 drops of the tincture.

Toxicity: The herb is thought to be low in toxicity but may cause dermatitis. The emodin in large doses could cause nausea, vomiting, diarrhea, and cramping.

Comments: Other than a slight stimulant action by the emodin, there does not appear to be any basis for its use to remove bladder stones.

References: 3, 17, 36, 42

Lady's Slipper
(Cypripedium pubescens)

Known Principles: Besides tannins and resin, lady's slipper also contains a volatile oil and a volatile acid.

Mode of Action: The tannins are protein precipitants and the volatile oil is a mucous membrane irritant, carminative, and diaphoretic.

Alleged Uses: The dried roots and rhizomes are recommended as a sedative, nerve "restorative," remedy for excitability, diaphoretic, and antispasmodic.

Toxicity: The stems and leaves possess glandular hairs that will produce irritation on the body if handled. This dermatitis resembles that of poison ivy and may occur 8–12 hours after handling the plant.

Comments: It is unlikely that enough of the volatile oil is ingested to cause significant drowsiness. If this were so, stomach upset should also be present.

References: 3, 9, 36

Lemongrass
(Cymbopogon citracus)

Known Principles: Lemongrass contains the aldehyde citronellal, methyl heptenone, terpenes, and terpene alcohols.

Mode of Action: The volatile oil in lemongrass has some pesticide activity but is less effective than malathion. The insect-repellent properties are attributed to the methyl heptenone.

Alleged Uses: Lemongrass is commonly recommended in herbals as a carminative, perfume, and insect repellent.

Toxicity: The dangers of lemongrass are similar to those of other volatile oils. There may be some central nervous system depression or mucous membrane irritation if the agent is taken in sufficient quantities. No cases of serious poisoning have been reported.

References: 1, 16, 17

Leopard's Bane
(Arnica montana)
(Mountain tobacco, Wolf's Bane)

Known Principles: Besides choline, *Arnica* contains 0.5–1% volatile oil consisting of dimethyl ether of thymohydroquinone. There is also arnidendiol (found in dandelion flowers), angelic and formic acid, fatty acids, and two unidentified substances that affect the cardiovascular system.

Mode of Action: The active principles are irritants that produce a violent toxic gastroenteritis, pulse abnormalities, nervous change, intense muscular weakness, cardiovascular collapse, and death. It is used topically as a counterirritant.

Alleged Uses: Today this herb is rarely used by physicians, but it is still a domestic remedy to provide a counterirritant effect on strains and bruises. It has also seen use against palsies and other illnesses, but there is little information on its actions or usefulness concerning these treatments. The dried flowers are thought to be bacteriocidal. Normal doses are 60–200 mg of the flowers and 0.5 mls of the tincture.

Toxicity: Many of the toxic symptoms are listed above. Fatally poisoned persons have had burning pain of the stomach, vomiting, diarrhea, and coma. In some cases the central nervous system depressant effects predominate with very little early gastroenteritis. An overdose of the tincture is serious, but most likely not fatal.

Comments: Do not confuse this plant with either Wolf's Bane (*Aconitum* spp., monkshood), or Indian tobacco (*Lobelia* spp.).

References: 2, 6, 17

Licorice
(*Glycyrrhiza glabra*)

Known Principles: Licorice contains glycyrrhizin (5–10%), starch (29%), sugar, gum, protein, resin, fat (0.8%), asparagine (2–4%), and traces of tannin, a yellow dye, a volatile oil, and pentacyclic terpenes.

Mode of Action: Licorice has mild mineralocorticoid properties, spasmolytic properties, and estrogenic properties. The terpene has a structure resembling that of steroids. The plant also contains a hemolytically active saponin in the inner bark.

Alleged Uses: Licorice root is used primarily as a demulcent and emollient. Doses are 1–4 teaspoons of the fluid extract or ½–1 teaspoons of the powdered root.

Toxicity: Licorice is relatively safe but large amounts deplete potassium, cause sodium retention, and result in electrolyte imbalance, hypertension, and edema.

Comments: Patients with any preexisting hypertension or other cardiovascular disease should avoid the use of licorice root, as it is likely to aggravate their conditions.

References: 1, 3, 6, 17

Life Root
(Senecio vulgaris, S. aureus) (Groundsel)

Known Principles: *Senecio* contains a number of pyrrolizidine alkaloids. More than 40 have been identified from various *Senecio* species.

Mode of Action: These alkaloids produce hypertensive pulmonary vascular disease. Some have been shown to decrease carcinosarcoma in mice, and others show antileukemic activity in subhepatotoxic levels. The herb appears to have low therapeutic value.

Alleged Uses: Herbalists most often use this agent for irregularities of the menses, e.g., dysmenorrhea, menorrhagia, atonic leukorrhea, and other disturbances of the pelvic organs. It has also been used to hasten delayed childbirth.

Toxicity: The pyrrolizidine alkaloids have produced toxic necrosis of the liver. *Senecio* is most toxic in its young stages. North American varieties seem not to be as toxic as some species grown elsewhere. *S. aureus* appears to be less toxic than other members of this group.

Comments: Since this herb appears to have little effect on the uterus, there appears to be little basis for current recommended uses.

References: 1, 2, 3, 11, 17, 36, 37, 39

Lily-of-the-Valley
(*Convallaria majalis*)

Known Principles: Lily-of-the-valley contains several crystalline glycosides usually called convallarin and convallamarin, but there are other names.

Mode of Action: These alkaloids have an action on the heart similar to digitalis but have little cumulative tendency and are more active as a diuretic. Convallatoxin is the primary cardioactive material, being 10 times as active as digitoxin and 16 times as active on test animal hearts. One-tenth gm of *Convallaria* is equal in potency to 12 digitalis units. Clinical trials have shown *Convallaria* to be inferior to digitalis when clinical improvement is measured.

Alleged Uses: This herb is often recommended for "weak" hearts and to improve the circulation. The dried roots and rhizomes are used in tea or made into a tincture.

Toxicity: Overdoses of *convallaria* cause nausea, vomiting, violent purging, and cardiac arrthymias. Symptoms usually occur more rapidly than if digitalis (foxglove) were ingested. Skin rashes have also been reported after handling the plant.

Comments: This is a potentially very dangerous agent and should not be taken without a physician's knowledge and advice.

References: 1, 2, 3, 11, 17, 36

Linden Flowers
(*Tilia europea*) (Lime Tree)

Known Principles: Lime's primary constituents are tannins and a volatile oil.

Mode of Action: This plant is mildly astringent and has spasmolytic and diaphoretic properties, most likely due to the volatile oil.

Alleged Uses: Lime is most often recommended as a chronic cough remedy with expectorant properties. The dried flowers are what is used to make teas and tinctures. Normal dose of the tincture is 15–40 drops.

Toxicity: Linden is not considered to be highly toxic. If the flowers used in the preparation are too old, they may cause drowsiness.

References: 1, 6, 36

Lobelia
(*Lobelia inflata*)

Known Principles: The active ingredient is lobeline. Also present are lobelidine, lobelanine, nor-lobelaine, lobelanidine, nor-lobelanidine, lobinine, and isolobenine. The alkaloid content ranges from 0.13– 0.63% and up to one-half of the total alkaloid content may be lobeline. Some studies have shown that lobelia contains at least 14 different types of piperidine alkaloids.

Mode of Action: The action of lobeline is much like nicotine. Lobeline is a primary stimulant and a secondary depressant to the autonomic ganglia. It also exerts a stimulating effect on certain medullary centers, especially the emetic center.

Alleged Uses: Lobelia is recommended by herbalists as an expectorant, an asthma treatment, or an emetic. Usual dose may be as high as 100 mg. The leaves and seed capsule may be chewed to produce giddiness, headache, and general tremors.

Toxicity: Lobelia is a powerful poison and should not be used in home remedies since dosing errors would have serious consequences. Toxic manifestations start with nausea and vomiting, progress through stupor, tremors, and paralysis, and terminate with convulsions, coma, and death. In one study by Cooper, it was reported that as little as 50 mg of dried herb or 1 ml of tincture of lobelia has produced alarming symptoms in some people. Therefore, individuals may become poisoned on even "therapeutic" amounts.

Comments: Lobelia is one of the constituents of "legal grass" that has been advertised by some "dope magazines." This mixture is advertised for weight loss, which may actually occur, since most individuals do not eat much while nauseated.

References: 1, 3, 4, 5, 6, 17, 30

Malabar Nut Tree
(Adhatoda vasica) (Vasaka)

Known Principles: The primary ingredients in malabar nut tree are adhatodic acid and the alkaloid vasicine. Vasicine appears to be identical to another plant alkaloid called peganine.

Mode of Action: Studies in experimental animals have shown that vasicine induces a mild but persistent dilation of the bronchi. There is also an unidentified substance that is active against tubercle bacilli.

Alleged Uses: Both the fresh and dried leaves have long been used as a mucolytic agent for the treatment of colds, bronchitis, asthma, and other respiratory diseases. Today it is most often recommended as an expectorant. The usual dose is 1–2 gms of the dried leaves.

Toxicity: Toxicity data on this plant are scanty. Large doses irritate the bowels and will cause nausea, vomiting, and diarrhea. It is claimed that this herb will not harm higher animals, but only lower animals and plants. This claim is not substantiated by fact.

References: 1, 6, 9, 16, 17

Male Fern
(Dryopteris filix-mass) *(Dryopteris* spp.)
(Aspidium)

Known Principles: These ferns contain 6.5–15% of an oleoresin that contains the filmaron and filicic acid. Other agents said to be in the oleoresin include aspidinin, albaspidin, aspidin, aspidinol, and flavaspininic acid. Besides the oleoresin, a volatile oil, sugar, starch, several resins, wax, and tannins have been found.

Mode of Action: The active ingredient appears to be the oleoresin, especially the filmaron and filicic acid. These agents are anthelmintic. Aspidinol appears to have some phenolic properties. Some components of other *Dryopteris* species have been shown to be muscle poisons.

Alleged Uses: The rhizomes, frondal bases, and apical buds are the parts used for their anthelmintic properties. Since the powdered plant tends to lose its potency rapidly, the stable oleoresin is usually the pharmaceutical preparation.

Toxicity: The plant may cause symptoms in even therapeutic doses. Most commonly seen are nausea, vomiting, cramping, headache, dyspnea, albuminuria, and bilirubinuria. Severe poisonings result in loss of reflexes, optic neuritis, impairment of vision, temporary or permanent blindness, coma, convulsions, and death due to cardiac or respiratory failure.

Comments: This agent is generally contraindicated with pregnancy, old or debilitated patients, anemia, gastrointestinal ulceration, or impaired cardiac, hepatic, or renal function.

References: 1, 2, 17, 45

Mandrake, American
(Podophyllum peltatum) (Mayapple)

Known Principles: Mandrake has 3.5–6% ligan glycosides composing a resin. These glycosides are podophyllotoxin, alpha-peltatin, and beta-peltatin.

Mode of Action: The ligan glycosides owe their antimitotic and purgative properties to a lactone ring in the trans configuration. Treatment with mild alkali changes the formation to cis and renders it inactive.

Alleged Uses: This agent is recommended for treatment of constipation and atonic bowel. It has also seen use as a "paint" for venereal and other warts.

Toxicity: The resin is strongly irritating to skin and mucous membranes. Symptoms may occur from eating green fruit or eating or handling foliage or roots. Severe cases may result in drowsiness, lethargy, or unconsciousness in 12–24 hours.

Comments: This should not be confused with *Mandragora*, called mandrake by the Greeks and Asiatics.

References: 1, 3, 7, 8, 29

Mandrake
(*Mandragora officanarum*) (Satan's Apple)

Known Principles: This herb contains hyoscyamine, scopolamine, mandragorin, and smaller amounts of minor alkaloids.

Mode of Action: This poisonous narcotic is similar to belladonna in its action and is a parasympatholytic. It has little effect on blood vessels; in larger amounts it will increase heart rate, dilate pupils, cause dryness of the mouth, urinary retention, and hallucinations, and reduce intestinal peristalis.

Alleged Uses: Mandrake has many and varied recommended uses. These include use as a pain killer, a sedative, an aphrodisiac, and a death simulation, as well as treatment for ulcers, skin sores, skin diseases, and hemorrhoids. This plant has even been recommended as a demonic, emetic, purgative, and anesthetic.

Toxicity: This is a product that will produce anticholinergic symptoms as listed above. Death is usually a result of heart rhythm abnormalities.

Comments: This plant is a member of the nightshade family. It is thought to have magical properties. This plant should not be confused with the American mandrake (*Podophyllum*). Some say the leaves are harmless, but the alkaloids are present in all parts of the plant.

References: 2, 6, 11, 17, 46

Marshmallow plant
(*Althea officinalis*)

Known Principles: *Althea* averages 37% starch, 25–35% mucilage, 11% pectin, 11% sugar, 1.25% fat, and 2% asparagine.

Mode of Action: The plant has only demulcent and emollient actions.

Alleged Uses: The part of the plant most commonly used is the root. It is used in a decoction for inflammation of mucous membranes and as a demulcent. The roots, leaves, and flowers are employed as a poultice and excipient in pills.

Toxicity: None

Comments: Should not be harmful unless patient has a bowel disorder or obstruction.

References: 1, 2, 17

Maté
(Ilex paraguariensis St. Hill)

Known Principles: The primary ingredient is caffeine, up to 2%.

Mode of Action: Caffeine is a known central nervous system stimulant, and in large doses, a diuretic.

Alleged Uses: The dried leaves have been used as a tea to produce hallucinations. It has also been recommended as a laxative, diuretic, and diaphoretic.

Toxicity: Caffeine is generally considered to be low in toxicity, but large amounts, or excessive use, may cause symptoms of nervousness, insomnia, increased heart rate, or aggravation of peptic ulcers.

Comments: Care should be taken if this product is taken frequently by patients with high blood pressure, heart disease, ulcers, or hyperactivity.

References: 29, 30

Matricaria
(Matricaria chamomilla)
(Hungarian or German Chamomile)

Known Principles: All parts of the plant are active, but the flower heads are the only parts used officially. They contain 0.3–0.5% of a volatile oil composed of azulene, sesquiterpenes, sesquiterpene alcohol, paraffin hydrocarbons, umbelliferone methyl ether (methylcoumarin), furfural, and a fatty acid. They also contain alphabisabolol, which gives the oil its blue color. Tannins and up to 3% glycosides have also been demonstrated.

Mode of Action: The alpha-bisabolol was found to have some anti-inflammatory action in rats. The glycoside affects smooth muscle, and in large doses may paralyze it. Ventricular catheterization studies on heart patients given the tea found no significant cardiac effects. There was a marked drowsiness seen, since most of the patients fell asleep within 10 minutes of receiving the tea. The oil is irritating enough to be used as a counterirritant for treating bruises and contusions.

Alleged Uses: Some European physicians have recommended its use as a antispasmodic and anthelmintic, but this practice is not common in the U.S. Matricaria has found some use as a mild tonic-sedative like *Anthemis* (Roman chamomile). It has been recommended as a carminative, but is not very effective. Its pineapplelike odor has made it useful in flavoring ice cream, candy, and liqueurs.

Toxicity: The only reported symptoms, if excessive amounts are ingested, are nausea and vomiting, with moderate sedation. The plant has also caused dermatitis.

References: 1, 2, 17, 24

May Flower
(*Anemone pulsatilla*)

Known Principles: This plant contains anemone camphor, volatile oil, tannins, and ranunculin.

Mode of Action: The ranunculin (anemonin) is broken down to protoanemonin, a strong mucous membrane irritant. The tannins are astringents and the volatile oil an expectorant.

Alleged Uses: According to herbalists, this herb is useful in treating disorders of menstruation and spermatorrhea. It is supposed to lessen sexual excitement but increase sexual strength. Recommended dose is 1–3 drops of the tincture every 2–3 hours.

Toxicity: The toxic chemical is ranunculin. Individuals may get dermatitis from handling the plant. If ingested in quantity, it may produce a burning sensation of the mouth and throat, colic, gastrointestinal pain, and even kidney damage. Symptoms have been reported after eating the flower in salad. The toxicity is thought to be lost on drying or cooking.

Comments: The recommendations are rather nonspecific, and a gastrointestinal irritant is likely to decrease sexual excitement, but it does not appear to have any definite effect on the sexual organs.

References: 9, 36

Milkweed

(*Asclepias* spp.) (Blood-flower, many other common names, depending on the species)

Known Principles: This plant contains asclepiadin, asclepion (a bitter), galitoxin, and another similar resin, volatile oils, and some other glycoside.

Mode of Action: Although the glycosides are known to have cardiac action, most activity seems to come from the resin principles. There appears to be an expectorant and diaphoretic action of small to normal doses. Larger amounts cause vomiting and catharsis. There have been some reports that it has diuretic and estrogenic actions.

Alleged Uses: The various parts of the plant have been made into both tea and fluid extract. It is often used for treating bronchitis and rheumatism. Some use the young tender leaves as a pot herb. The normal dose is 1–4 mls of the fluid extract.

Toxicity: Many of the species are known to be poisonous. All parts of the plant are toxic. Many of the case reports concern animals, but human poisonings have been reported. Typical symptoms include gastrointestinal upset, diarrhea, central nervous system depression, anorexia, ataxia, kidney and liver damage, and seizures. Symptom onset is usually delayed a couple of hours after the ingestion.

References: 3, 17, 16, 17, 34

Milkwort
(Polygala vulgaris, P. senega)

Known Principles: Various members of the *Polygala* family contain glycosidal saponins.

Mode of Action: The glycosidal saponins are not well-absorbed orally, but they are strong intestinal irritants that give rise to reflex secretion of mucus in the bronchioles. This herb is classed as a stimulant, expectorant, possible diuretic and diaphoretic, and emetic.

Alleged Uses: Milkwort is often recommended as a lactation acid. Generally, it is used with mitchella to stimulate lactation before pregnancy. Indians believe it to be a cure for snakebite. Other recommendations include treatment of gout, pleurisy, rheumatism, hives, and croup, and to create vomiting and catharsis. Usually 9 drops of the tincture is the recommended dose.

Toxicity: Excessive amounts may produce violent vomiting and purging, as well as central nervous system depression. Cases are similar to other saponin poisonings.

Comments: In small amounts this herb could be an expectorant or laxative. It appears to have little effect on lactation, and there are safer agents to use for inducing emesis.

References: 6, 36, 39

Mistletoe
(*Phoradendron* spp.)

Known Principles: Mistletoe contains several stimulant amines, including tyramine and beta phenylethylamine.

Mode of Action: The amines stimulate the heart and central nervous system, increase blood pressure, and cause contraction of intestinal and uterine smooth muscle. They are also vasodilators but this action is usually delayed and has a maximal effect 3–4 days after administration of mistletoe.

Alleged Uses: Mistletoe was used by Indians and pioneers as a oxytoxic agent to arrest postpartum hemorrhage. It has also been used in hysteria and in the treatment of cholera. Mistletoe has been recommended as a sedative and as a treatment for high blood pressure, but there is no basis in fact for these uses. The amines would seem to have the exact opposite actions.

Toxicity: Mistletoe contains toxic amines and proteins that may cause gastrointestinal upset. There have been both animal and human deaths caused from mistletoe.

Symptoms commonly noted with overdose include slow heart rate, convulsions, hallucinations, increased blood pressure, and cardiovascular collapse. Death has been reported as late as 10 hours after ingestion. One to two berries may be a significantly toxic dose.

Comments: Since this plant is used as a common Christmas decoration, extreme care should be taken to keep it out of the reach of children. Homemade teas made from mistletoe berries may be extremely dangerous.

References: 3, 10, 11, 16, 17, 23

Monkshood
(Aconitum napellus, Aconitum spp.)

Known Principles: Monkshood contains a number of very toxic alkaloids (0.3–1%). The concentration of the various alkaloids varies considerably between various species, but usually approximately 0.2% aconitine is found, along with traces of picratonitine, aconine, benzoylamine, and neopelline, to name just a few.

Mode of Action: The alkaloids in monkshood first stimulate, then depress both central and peripheral nerves. Its nervous activity resembles that of protoveratrine in some respects, while its cardiovascular effects are similar to quinidine. Topically it is a local irritant, counterirritant, and paralizant to the peripheral sensory nerves.

Alleged Uses: Monkshood has been widely recommended in homeopathic medicine. It has been used to decrease the action of the heart, to decrease blood pressure, to decrease temperature (most likely due to decreased blood pressure, which reflexively increases sweating), and to treat various neuralgias and nervous disorders. It is sometimes recommended as a local anesthetic.

Toxicity: This herb is very poisonous. Human poisonings have occurred as a result of the leaves being mistaken for wild parsley, or the roots for horseradish. Poisoning may also result as a misuse of the herb as a medication. Symptoms include an initial tingling or burning sensation of the lips and tongue, followed by numbness. This may progress to difficulty in swallowing, speech difficulty, nausea, and vomiting, restlessness, irritability, confusion, and intense headache. Vision may be blurred or doubled, breathing slowed, and pupils become pinpoint. Death may ensue as early as a few minutes after ingestion or as late as 4 days. Even after successful management, patients exhibit exhaustion and sensory disturbances for a long time. The lethal human dose is around 5 mg of the pure alkaloids or a teaspoonful of the root.

Comments: This agent has been used as a poison for a long time. Primitives used it as an arrow poison. The homeopathic preparation called aconite is very hard to standardize as to physiological activity. Thus, it is somewhat dangerous to use, even for those who know what they are doing.

References: 1, 2, 3, 5, 7, 8, 11, 17, 36

Mormon Tea
(*Ephedra nevadensis, E. trifurca*)

Known Principles: This plant belongs to a larger group, all of which contain the chemical ephedrine. The actual concentration of ephedrine in Mormon tea has not been determined.

Mode of Action: Ephedrine is a stimulant. In sufficient amounts it will increase blood pressure, increase heart rate, and serve as a general nervous stimulant.

Alleged Uses: The settlers, Indians, and Mexicans have used Mormon tea as a stimulant drink. It has also been used as treatment for asthma, rheumatism, syphilis, various fevers, and nasal congestion.

Toxicity: Since Mormon tea contains a stimulant, individuals with high blood pressure, heart abnormalities or diabetes should take care when using this product. Since the concentration of ephedrine in Mormon tea is still unknown, the extent of danger involved with drinking the tea is somewhat in question. However, care should be exercised when using this product.

References: 16, 22, 30

Morning Glory
(*Ipomoea purpurea*)

Known Principles: Most members of the *Ipomoea* family contain 6.5–22% irritant resin. Morning glory also has up to 0.05% amides of lysergic acid, some scopoletin, a dihydroxycinnamic acid, a volatile oil and cetyl alcohol.

Mode of Action: The plant is primarily a purgative and hallucinogen. The cathartic action lies in the irritant properties of the resin.

Alleged Uses: Previously this plant was used solely for its purgative properties. When the amines of lysergic acid were found, morning glory seeds were used extensively for their hallucinogenic properties.

Toxicity: Symptoms of overdose include nausea, catharsis, blurred or disturbed vision, mental confusion, hallucinations, or coma. Fifty or more seeds are needed to have a marijuanalike effect.

Comments: Other members of the *Ipomoea* family are used primarily for their cathartic effect. One common name applies to the irritant resin common to this group: scammony resin. Not all members of *Ipomoea* have the toxic resin. *I. leptophylla* (bush morning glory) is said to be edible and good. Care should be taken to correctly identify a species if one is going to use it as a survival food.

References: 2, 3, 13, 17, 21

Mountain Ash

(*Sorbus aucuparia*) (Rowan Tree)

Known Principles: The fruits of this tree contain the sugar sorbose, sorbitol, and sorbic acid. They also have malic acid and 22% fixed oil.

Mode of Action: Sorbitol is a humectant and sweetener as well as an osmotic diuretic and cathartic. The berries are very slow fermenting, and therefore are stored more easily than some other berries.

Alleged Uses: The fruits and seeds are used in the treatment of scurvy and as an infusion for the treatment of hemorrhoids. They also are often used as a demulcent for various gastrointestinal disorders.

Toxicity: Very little toxicity is expected. The berries are edible. Excessive amounts could cause diarrhea.

Comments: At one time McNeil Laboratories had a compound called Sorparin, which was composed of sorbitol and used in the treatment of gall bladder irritation and digestive upset.

References: 2, 3, 17, 26

Mulberry
(*Morus rubra, Morus* spp.)

Known Principles: Although mulberry is known to have some physiologic activity, the chemical responsible for this is unknown.

Mode of Action: Because the active principles are unknown, the mechanisms by which it produces its effects are also unknown.

Alleged Uses: The berries are often crushed into a juice used in fever reductions, to induce drowsiness, and to serve as a laxative. The inner bark is made into a tea that is used as a laxative. The outer bark is recommended as an anthelmintic. Indians rubbed the sap on their skin for prevention of ringworm.

Toxicity: The sap from leaves and stems, as well as the unripe fruit, are known to be toxic. Symptoms most often seen are stomach irritation, central nervous system stimulation, and hallucination. The ripe berries appear to be harmless.

References: 3, 39, 52

Mullein
(Verbascum thapsiforme, V. phlomoides, V. thapsus)

Known Principles: Leaves contain several saponins. but most likely their action is too slight for physiologic action.

Mode of Action: It is doubtful whether it has any therapeutic value other than as a demulcent.

Alleged Uses: Mullein leaves have a mucilaginous and slightly bitter taste. Dried leaves have been smoked for relief of upper respiratory tract irritation. Other uses include external application for sunburn, hemorrhoids, and abraded skin or mucous membranes, as well as orally for a large variety of chest pains. Dose is 4–8 mls of the fluid extract.

Toxicity: There are no reports of toxic ingestions, probably because of low pharmacologic action.

References: 1, 3, 17

Myrrh
(Commiphora molmol)

Known Principles: Myrrh contains 25–45% resin, 55–60% gum, 7–17% volatile oil with traces of free acetic, formic, and myrrholic acids.

Mode of Action: Like other oleoresins, myrrh is locally stimulating and may perhaps stimulate peristalsis. It is an astringent to mucous membranes. Orally, it also has a carminative action.

Alleged Uses: It is primarily used as a constituent of perfumes and incenses. It has been used as a mild cathartic and for dyspepsia. Its astringency was used in a tincture intended for a mouthwash. Normal dose of the herb is 0.3–1.2 gms.

Toxicity: Its toxicology is much like that of the other volatile oils. In significant amounts one might expect some central nervous system depression initially, then later CNS stimulation to convulsions. Aspiration is unlikely in the form in which it is usually consumed, but if the volatile oil were distilled or concentrated, then it would be a significant hazard.

Comments: Myrrh was an ingredient in embalming fluids of the Egyptians.

References: 1, 17

Myrtle
(*Myrtus communis*)

Known Principles: The primary ingredient is a volatile oil called myrol (also called gelomyrotol). This oil consists primarily of eucalyptol and d-pinene.

Mode of Action: Specific information is lacking, but eucalyptol and d-pinene are both mucous membrane·irritants and in large amounts may produce CNS depression or convulsions.

Alleged Uses: The leaves are used to make an infusion for treatment of stomatitis, or as a gargle. It has also been recommended for bronchitis and cystitis. Nonmedically it is used as a condiment, flavor, or essence in perfumes.

Toxicity: No toxic reports are available, but the potential for coma, convulsions, and kidney damage exists. The hazard must not be great, since there are no reports.

References: 9, 24, 45

Nutmeg
(*Myristica fragrans*)

Known Principles: The fixed oil (25–40%), starch, and protein have little activity. The volatile oil (5–15%) consists of myristicin, elemicin, eugenol, isoeugenol, methyleugenol, methylisoeugenol, and methoxyeugenol.

Mode of Action: The volatile oil has carminative properties. Myristicin was thought to be the pharmacologically active agent but it, when given alone, does not produce the same effects as whole nutmeg. The hallucinogenic actions may be due to conversion of the myristicin to the psychoactive amine MMDA, and/or the elemicin being similarly converted to TMA.

Alleged Uses: Besides its abuse as an hallucinogen and its use as a spice, nutmeg has also been recommended for treatment of digestive disorders, rheumatism, cholera, and as an emmenagogue, abortifacient, and aphrodisiac.

Toxicity: As little as 5–15 gms (1–3 tsp.) may, within 3–6 hours, produce symptoms of nausea, vomiting, decreased body temperature, weak pulse and a feeling of pressure on the chest. From 6–12 hours after ingestion one may experience alternating periods of drowsiness and hallucination. Often there is a feeling of impending doom. Usually recovery is within 24 hours, but symptoms may last several days, including headache and dizziness.

Comments: This is not recommended as a hallucinogen. The effects are quite unpleasant.

References: 7, 30

Oak Bark
(Quercus spp.)

Known Principles: Oak bark contains 15–20% quercitannic acid.

Mode of Action: These tannins are protein precipitants and astringents.

Alleged Uses: Oak bark has been used to treat diarrhea and hemorrhoids, and as a gargle for sore throats.

Toxicity: Overdosage may result in abdominal pains, constipation, thirst, diarrhea, and polyuria. The plant also causes dermatitis. Severe overdoses may lead to liver and kidney damage.

References: 3, 4, 5

Oats or Oats Beards
(Avena sativa)

Known Principles: The primary compounds in oats include starch, gluten, albumin, sugar, gum oil, salts, and another protein compound. The straw contains a saponin and avenin.

Mode of Action: The plant is primarily a nutrient, but it has been found that the pericarp of oats contains an amphorous alkaloid that acts as a stimulant of the motor ganglia and increases the excitability of muscle. It has been known to cause excitement in horses. The starch, gluten, and albumin make it useful as a demulcent as well.

Alleged Uses: Oats are claimed to be a natural tonic,

"naturalizer" to the sexual system, and a "youthafier." They are claimed to have antidepressant activity and to decrease dependence on nicotine and morphine. (Studies showing this are controversial.) Naturally, they are also used as a food source.

Toxicity: There have been no reports of toxicity and the hazards from oats are low.

Comments: The term "feeling his oats" refers to the proposed "stimulant" effect that oats has on some animals, like horses.

References: 1, 2, 6, 12, 23, 36

Ololiuqui
(*Rivea corymbosa*)

Known Principles: This morning glory-type plant contains approximately 0.01% of five related LSD-like alkaloids. These include D-isolysergic acid amide, D-lysergic acid amide, chanoclavine, elymoclavine, and lysergol.

Mode of Action: The primary effect of this plant is to produce CNS depression and hallucination. As little as 1–2 mg of the alkaloid will produce psychomimetic effects.

Alleged Uses: Although the Mexican Indians still use the plant in magico-religious services, the primary use outside this group is abuse. It has no real medical importance.

Toxicity: To produce a marijuanalike effect, 50 or more seeds are needed. Overdoses produce symptoms of nausea, vomiting, blurred vision, confusion, incoordination, stupor, hallucinations and coma. There is great variability in the type of central nervous system effect seen with this plant. It varies not only between users, but between times used by the same abuser.

Comments: The brown seeds are often called *badah* by the Indians.

References: 1, 2, 3, 7, 16

Papaya
(*Carica papaya*)

Known Principles: Papaya contains the digestive enzyme papain. This enzyme is similar to pepsin and contains various proteolytic enzymes such as peptidase, and rennin-like coagulating enzymes, an amylolytic enzyme, and an enzyme that has a weak action on fats. This enzyme functions in acid, alkaline, and neutral media. The seeds contain a glycoside, caricin, and myrosin. These two compounds, when mixed, produce a mustardlike odor. The alkaloid carpine has also been found in the leaves. There are also appreciable amounts of vitamins C and E.

Mode of Action: The enzyme papain is a digestant. It is used both internally and externally. It also liberates histamine from the tissues. The alkaloid carpine has been shown to decrease heart rate and decrease central nervous system activity, and is an active amebicide.

Alleged Uses: Papaya's primary nonmedical use is as a meat tenderizer. Medically, it has been used to liquify excessive mucus in the mouth and stomach. The inner bark has been used for sore teeth, while the latex has been employed as an amebicide in Central America.

Toxicity: Papaya may be a strong allergen. There have been several cases where pharmacists who have worked with a product have developed a strong allergy to papaya. Other dangers include a possible destruction of esophageal wall with perforation if large amounts have been used.

References: 2, 3, 16, 17, 23

Parsley
(*Petroselinum sativum*)

Known Principles: All parts of parsley contain a volatile oil that gives its fragrance. This volatile oil is composed of a hydrocarbon, which is probably a pinene, and apiol. It also contains a flavone gylcoside called apiin. The apiol is called parsley camphor.

Mode of Action: A 1910 study involving apiol stated that it produced a decrease in blood pressure, a decrease in pulse rate, muscle weakness followed by paralysis, and convulsions. Postmortem studies showed significant lung congestion. Another study in 1908 showed apiol produced fatty degeneration of the liver in laboratory animals; it also produced muscle weakness.

Alleged Uses: Both the roots and the fuits (commonly called seeds) are used for medicinal purposes. Primary recommendation involve treatment for dysmenorrhea and other uterine disorders. It has even found some use as an abortifacient. It has also been recommended as a diuretic and as an aid in inflammation of the kidneys. However, in one study where 37 women were using the drug, one side effect noted was polyneuritis. There seem to be few concrete data to substantiate any of the claims. A normal dose of the root is around 2 gms, whereas the oil itself (apiol) is given in doses of 0.3–1 ml.

Toxicity: Although a scientific basis for its action on uterine muscle or kidney irritation has not been substantiated by scientific fact, that is not to say that it is without pharmacologic action. This substance, especially the oil, may be very dangerous if taken in inappropriate amounts. One case involves a pregnant woman who took 6 gms of the oil within a 48-hour period, then experienced dizziness, nausea, vomiting, uticaria, swollen liver, and mild icterus.

References: 2, 17

Partridgeberry
(*Mitchella repens*) (Squaw Vine)

Known Principles: Partridgeberry contains resin, wax, mucilage, dextrin, and what appear to be saponins.

Mode of Action: The pharmacology is not well worked out. It appears to be a diuretic and astringent. There may be gastrointestinal irritation due to the "saponin" component.

Alleged Uses: This herb is commonly recommended to ensure proper fetal development during pregnancy, to ease parturition, and to aid in developing lactation. It has also been recommended for insomnia, to decrease diarrhea, and to reduce edema. Herbalists say it resembles pipsissewa in action and is often substituted for it.

Toxicity: There have been no cases of toxicity reported.

Comments: It seems unlikely to have any action except as an astringent for diarrhea.

References: 6, 9, 36, 39

Passion Flower
(*Passiflora caerulea*)

Known Principles: The immature seeds, roots, and leaves contain cyanogenic glycosides. The leaves and stem also contain the alkaloids harmine, harman, harmol, and harmaline.

Mode of Action: The reported pharmacologic action of this agent is somewhat confusing in that it acts as a depressant of the spinal cord but increases the rate of respiration. It has very little effect on the circulation. Both harmine and harmaline are hallucinogenic alkaloids. Harmaline also has a marked central nervous system effect, including convulsion, motor paralysis, depression, and decreased body temperature.

Alleged Uses: The flowers and fruiting tops of this plant are taken in an effort to treat headaches, epilepsy, convulsions, and sleeplessness, and as a nerve tonic. Doses range from 200 mgs to 10 gms, or 10–20 minims of the fluid extract. Smoking passion flower is supposed to give a marijuanalike high, and the tea supposedly acts as a tranquilizer.

Toxicity: The plant may be toxic due to cyanogenic glycosides; however, no cases of cyanide poisoning have been reported from its use. If as little as 200 mgs of the alkaloid harmaline were to be ingested, such serious symptoms as convulsion, motor paralysis, marked central nervous system depression, a decrease in body temperature and a fall in blood pressure might result. There may also be respiratory paralysis or a decrease in strength of heart muscle.

References: 3, 5, 6, 17, 30

Peach
(*Prunus persica,* or other *Prunus* spp.)

Known Principles: All parts of the peach contain cyanide, but the kernels are especially rich. The leaves yield volatile oil with distillation. Phloretin has also been found in peach.

Mode of Action: Phloretin is an antibiotic that has been tested sucessfully against Gram-positive and Gram-negative bacteria. The volatile oil is likely to be irritant enough to serve as a carminative and gastrointestinal irritant.

Alleged Uses: Indians made a tea from the bark. The bark and root have been used as an antibiotic. The leaves, formerly thought to be an anthelmintic, are now used primarily as a laxative.

Toxicity: Animals have died from eating the leaves. The seed kernels, if ingested, have also caused serious cyanide poisoning in humans. All parts are potentially dangerous if eaten in sufficient quantities.

Comments: The quantity of cyanide available in *Prunus* species varies by the species, time of year, and climate condition. Although many individuals ingest peach kernels without harmful effects, there is still significant danger since the amount of cyanide per kernel may vary even between trees. Care should be exercised in using this plant for medicinal purposes.

References: 11, 16, 17

Pellitory
(Anacyclus pyrethrum)

Known Principles: Only known active substance is pellitorine (N-isobutyl amide of 2, 6, decadienoic acid).

Mode of Action: The only demonstrated effect of pellitory is that it has insecticidal properties.

Alleged Uses: The two uses most commonly recommended are relief of dental pain or facial pain, and to increase the flow of saliva with its bitter taste.

Toxicity: There have not been many reports of toxicity, but it is an irritant that could cause strong gastrointestinal irritation.

Comments: This plant should not be confused with the chrysanthemum, which yields pryethrum.

References: 17

Pennyroyal
(Mentha pulegium)

Known Principles: Ingredients found in pennyroyal include a yellow or greenish-yellow oil containing not less than 85% of the ketone, puligone.

Mode of Action: During excretion the oil irritates kidneys and bladder and reflexively excites uterine contraction. As with other volatile oils, it is also a CNS depressant, mucous membrane irritant, and external rubefacient. The mucous membrane irritation induces a feeling of warmth and increased salivation.

Alleged Uses: Pennyroyal has a strong musklike odor and an aromatic flavor; thus it has been used as a flavoring agent. Some have recommended it as an abortifacient.

Toxicity: As little as 4 mls of the oil have produced convulsion. There have been serious poisonings when the agent was used as an abortifacient. Symptoms include nausea, vomiting, diarrhea, and CNS depression. Nerve depression may change to stimulation and convulsions with larger doses.

Comments: It has been recommended that pennyroyal oil be prohibited as a flavoring agent in Britain. It should not be used with any preexisting kidney disease.

References: 1, 17

Peppermint
(*Mentha piperita*)

Known Principles: The leaves are said to contain tannic acid. Also present is 0.4–1.25% volatile oil, consisting primarily of menthol, menthone, methyl acetate, and terpenes.

Mode of Action: The volatile oil is an irritant to mucous membranes, a carminative, and aromatic.

Alleged Uses: Peppermint is recommended as an aromatic stimulant for colic and cramps in children. It is also a commonly used flavor in both medical and nonmedical preparation. Leaves and flowering tops are used as a dried powder, volatile oil, or tincture.

Toxicity: Generally, peppermint is not considered a toxic risk. There have been allergic reactions to the menthol component of the oil, and ingestion of greater than 5–10 gms of the oil could cause profound drowsiness and vomiting.

References: 1, 2, 17, 36

Periwinkle
(*Catharanthus roseus,* also called *Vinca rosea*)

Known Principles: Periwinkle contains nearly 55 different *Vinca* alkaloids, including vinblastine, vinleurosine, vinrosidine, and vincristine. One needs nearly 500 kg of *Catharanthus* to provide 1 gm of vincristine.

Mode of Action: The active principles produce granulocytopenia and bone marrow depression.

Alleged Uses: In folklore it is used as an oral hypogylcemic agent. Today it is much more likely to be smoked to create hallucinations.

Toxicity: Toxic symptoms are varied. They include drowsiness, blurred vision, dry mouth, nausea, and ataxia. More serious problems include liver damage, psychosis, hallucination, coma, convulsions, and death. Its antineoplastic activity may create alopecia or serious bone marrow depression.

References: 16, 29

Pigweed
(*Chenopodium album, C. ambrosioides*)
(Goosefoot, Wild Spinach, American Wormseed)

Known Principles: Besides being a rich source of calcium, vitamin A and vitamin C, pigweed contains 1–2% volatile oil and some saponins in the roots. The oil is composed of 45–70% ascaridol (an unsaturated terpene peroxide), 15% cymene, 10% terpene, 1-limonene, d-camphor, and some other hydrocarbons.

Mode of Action: Ascaridol is the most active, if not the sole active agent in this plant. A concentration of 1/200 is antiseptic. Doses of 0.02 ml/kg of the oil decrease the blood pressure, heart rate, and central nervous system activity. Large doses in mammals produce spinal cord depression and produce death by respiratory paralysis. There is some decrease in gastric motility, leading to constipation. The substance is an irritant and will leave a burning sensation in the mouth and throat.

Alleged Uses: The plant has a strong, offensive odor. Although all parts may be used, only the fruit was official in the drug compendia. The drug has been recommended as an external poultice and as a treatment for arthritis, but its only real use is as an anthelmintic. Extreme caution must be taken when using the oil. The normal dose for an adult is 1 ml of the oil.

Toxicity: If this herb is used carelessly, fatalities may result. Mild intoxications are common. Symptoms of poisoning include nausea, vomiting, headache, tinnitis, drowsiness, deafness, decrease in visual acuity, decreased respiration, slowed heart rate, and gastric ulcers. This is not a plant to be used casually.

Comments: The ascaridol is a peroxide that explodes on heating. The oil should not be used in patients who have heart, liver, kidney, stomach, or intestinal disease.

References: 2, 17, 39, 52

Pipsissewa
(*Chimaphila* spp.)

Known Principles: The leaves contain various constituents, including chimaphilin, arbutin, ericolin, urson, tannins, pectic acid, chlorophyll, and minerals.

Mode of Action: This plant appears to have a weak diuretic action.

Alleged Uses: Pipsissewa leaves are used as an extract or infusion to treat dyspepsia or as a urinary antiseptic. It has an action similar to uva-ursi. The commonly administered dose is 2–6 gms.

Toxicity: The plant has caused dermatitis and its astringency may produce gastrointestinal disorders if taken in large amounts.

References: 3, 5, 6, 15, 17

Pitcher Plant
(*Sarracenia* spp.)

Known Principles: The active principles include an alkaloid, a resin, and a yellow dye.

Alleged Uses: Infusions, powders and fluid extracts of pitcher plant roots have been used as a laxative, stomach tonic, and diuretic. The dose is 1 teaspoon of the fluid extract. This preparation is bitter and slightly astringent.

Toxicity: There is no evidence that this plant is toxic in reasonable quantities.

References: 3, 5, 6

Pleurisy Root
(*Asclepias tuberosa*) (Butterfly Weed)

Known Principles: Agents found include asclepiadin, asclepion (a bitter), galitoxin and similar resins, a volatile oil, and some glycosides. Most of the activity lies with the resinoid principles.

Mode of Action: The resins appear to be strong mucous membrane irritants.

Alleged Uses: Pleurisy root is used as an emetic, cathartic, diaphoretic, and expectorant agent.

Toxicity: All parts are toxic, but especially the stems and leaves. Symptoms range from mild to severe gastrointestinal upset, central nervous system depression, muscle weakness, loss of appetite, diarrhea and staggering, to death by respiratory paralysis in one to several days.

Comments: The reasons for its systemic effects are as yet unknown.

References: 3

Pokeberry
(*Phytolacca americana*)

Known Principles: Pokeberries contain triterpene saponins (one is phytolaccigenin), mitogens, glycoproteins, asparagine, and an unidentified resin.

Mode of Action: The saponins are irritants, causing emesis and catharsis. The resin may be a CNS depressant.

Alleged Uses: Pokeberry has been recommended for chronic rheumatism, as an ingredient in an ointment with antiparasitic properties, and as a laxative. Only the laxative use has any basis in scientific fact. The dose as a cathartic is 60–300 mg.

Toxicity: This herb contains mitogens that may cause aberrations when absorbed through broken skin. It also causes a peripheral blood plasmacytosis. Ingestions cause nausea, vomiting, and diarrhea. The onset of diarrhea is usually slow, with onset two or more hours after ingestion. There may be either decreased heart rate or respiratory rate leading to death. The fruit is less toxic than the leaves, which are less toxic than the stems, which are less toxic than the roots.

Comments: This herb has been known to produce skin abrasions by simply handling of the roots. Poke is a common potherb in the South. Even though there is little of the toxin in the immature shoots and the toxin is destroyed by heat, use of poke as a potherb may be dangerous and is not recommended.

References: 1, 3, 9, 16

Pomegranate
(*Punica granatum*)

Known Principles: There is a mixture of tannins (22–28%) in all parts of the plant. The roots contain a mixture of four alkaloids called pelletierine. These alkaloids are pelletierine, pseudopelletierine, isopelletierine and methylisopelletierine.

Mode of Action: The fruit rinds and bark are very astringent. The pelletierine is an anthelmintic. The results of phar-

macology studies vary greatly when dealing with pelletierine. It seems that in large doses the pelletierine
could cause complete paralysis.

Alleged Uses: The fruits are edible, but the rind and bark are
used as an astringent. The alkaloids in the roots had
widespread use against tapeworm until less toxic substances were discovered.

Toxicity: Toxicity is chiefly of the pelletierine tannate. The
symptoms include muscle weakness, dizziness, and in
larger doses mydriasis, amblyopia, vomiting, and
diarrhea. Blindness, most likely due to inflammation of
the optic nerve, has occurred and occasionally been permanent.

References: 1, 2, 8, 17

Poplar Bud
(*Populus candicans*)

Known Principles: The buds contain a balsam-like resin, a
yellow volatile oil (primarily humulene), gallic acid, malic
acid, mannite, chrysin, tectochrysin, a fixed oil, and two
glycosides, salicin and populin. (Populin is salicin ben-
zoate.)

Mode of Action: The salicin has some antipyretic and
analgesic action. The resin yields a terpene to which
many of its therapeutic effects are attributed. It has an
action similar to turpentine.

Alleged Uses: The air-dried, closed winter leaf buds are used
both medically and nonmedically. There appears to be an
antioxidant present that makes it useful in preventing
rancidity in certain ointments. When used externally,
poplar is a mild counterirritant for muscle strain or

rheumatism. Internally, it is primarily a stimulant expectorant used for the cough of colds or bronchitis. It is an additive in several pharmaceutical preparations, including pine syrup.

Toxicity: There have been no reports of serious poisonings due to poplar, but skin rashes and pollen sensitizations are fairly common.

References: 2, 3, 7, 8, 9, 17

Prickly Ash
(Northern—*Xanthoxylum americanum*)
(Southern—*Xanthoxylum clava-herculus*)

Known Principles: Prickly ash contains 3–4% essential oil, a resin, berberine, and several related bases. Southern prickly ash contains asarinin, an acid amide, and herculin (which is an insecticide with actions similar to pyrethrins). Northern prickly ash has small quantities of alkaloids that have not been shown to be medically important. Xanthoxyletin and xanthyletin have been isolated in this species by investigators.

Mode of Action: Prickly ash does have carminative properties. Some species, when swallowed, give enough irritation to produce "heat" in the stomach, and promote diaphoresis. It appears the only therapeutic effect the fruit has is as a mild astringent and aromatic.

Alleged Uses: The bark, leaves, and fruits have all been recommended for use. Most herbalists use it as a gastric stimulant like capsicum; therefore it is suggested for many chronic gastrointestinal disorders, syphilis, scrofula, rheumatism, and arthritis.

Toxicity: Human poisonings have not been reported but it

has been suspected of livestock losses in several states. Data on toxicity are still unclear.

Comments: This herb is likely to be safely used as a carminative, but its use as an irritant in chronic bowel disorders should be avoided, and it would have little therapeutic value against arthritis or rheumatism.

References: 1, 2, 11, 17, 36

Prickly Poppy
(*Argemone mexicana*)

Known Principles: These plants contain a number of isoquinoline alkaloids such as protopine and berberine. The seeds also contain dihydrosanquinarine and sanquinarine.

Mode of Action: The alkaloids in the seeds have produced dilation of capillaries, resulting in leaking of fluids into the tissues. Although morphine and codeine are papaverine derivatives of isoquinoline alkaloids, there appears to be little central nervous system depressant effect from the above alkaloids.

Alleged Uses: Up to this point, one of the primary problems for humans has occurred when the seeds were mixed with home-grown grains. Now abuse is a new problem, with the plant being smoked in the hope of producing narcotic or euphoric effects. Comanche Indians are known to have applied an extract of the seeds to sore eyes.

Toxicity: Much of the toxic manifestations are well known because of animal data. As little as 1 ounce of seeds has produced symptoms in animals. These symptoms include nausea, vomiting, diarrhea, visual difficulties, swelling of the abdominal cavity, generalized edema, dizziness and fainting, coma, and cardiac toxicity. Humans may develop similar symptoms by eating the seeds directly or consuming contaminated milk products.

References: 2, 3, 11, 22, 26

Psyllium
(*Plantago psyllium*)

Known Principles: Psyllium contains primarily mucilage, a glycoside, and two acids.

Mode of Action: One gram of seeds will swell to 8–14 times its volume when placed in water. This property makes it very useful as a bulk laxative. It appears its action is purely mechanical, and the glycosides and acids have little or no pharmacologic effect.

Alleged Uses: The seeds of this plant are taken with water to alleviate constipation. The mucilage also has demulcent properties. Normal doses range from 4–5 gms.

Toxicity: There have been no serious reports of toxicity with this plant.

Comments: Individuals with bowel obstruction or bowel diseases should contact their physician before using this herb.

References: 1, 2, 7, 17

Red Clover
(*Trifolium* spp.)

Known Principles: The active principles, if any, are yet undescribed. Some phenolic substances and two glycosides have been discovered.

Mode of Action: As of yet, there is no evidence that these principles are physiologically active.

Alleged Uses: Red clover is claimed to be useful as an antispasmodic and expectorant. These claims have led to its use in its treatment of bronchitis and whooping cough. There is no evidence that its use in this manner is efficacious. The usual dose is 4 gms.

Toxicity: No toxic ingestions have been noted with this plant.

References: 17

Red Raspberry
(*Rubus strigosus* or *R. idaeus*)

Known Principles: Raspberries contain greater than 1.5% citric acid, as well as some tannins in the leaves, roots, and bark. Other active principles are yet unknown.

Mode of Action: Red raspberry has been shown in animals to relax the smooth muscle of the uterus and intestine.

Alleged Uses: A strong infusion of leaves and roots has been used to loosen the bowel. It has also found use as a remedy in menorrhagia and to regulate labor pains. Its astringency has made it of use in dysentery and as a gargle. The berries are, of course, edible.

Toxicity: There is no evidence of toxic ingestions from raspberry tea. However, since the leaves do contain tannins, chronic bowel irritation or kidney irritation is a possibility.

References: 1, 3, 16, 17

Rhatany
(Krameria triandra)

Known Principles: Besides 8–20% tannins, *Krameria* contains lignin, minute amounts of gum, starch, and a saccharine, and 8–9% krameric acid. Calcium oxalate and n-methyl-tyrosine have also been found.

Mode of Action: Rhatany has astringent properties similar to tannic acids and therefore is an active astringent. Claims that *Krameria* promotes epithelizations of wounds appear unsubstantiated, except as a protein precipitant.

Alleged Uses: Formerly rhatany was recommended for sore throat, hermorrhoids, chronic inflammations of the bowel, and diarrhea. It has even seen use against typhoid fever.

Toxicity: Tannic acids, being strongly astringent, may cause nausea, vomiting, and other types of gastrointestinal distress. Large amounts may also cause kidney damage. No human poisonings have been reported.

Comments: This agent could be harmful rather than beneficial in dealing with chronic bowel problems. It should never be taken without a physician's advice.

References: 1, 2, 17, 36

Rheumatism Root
(Dioscarea villosa) (Wild Yam Root)

Known Principles: Besides an acrid resin, *Dioscarea* contains a saponin (dioscin). The aglycone of dioscin (diosgenin) is a steroid base from which progesterone and cortisone have been synthesized.

Mode of Action: Dioscin is an extraordinary hemolytic agent. It is very toxic to both fish and amoeba. There also may be some expectorant and diuretic properties, but this still is unclear. It does not appear to have any of the antispasmodic properties claimed, and therefore would be of little use in treating biliary colic.

Alleged Uses: Rheumatism root has long been used as a domestic remedy for rheumatism. It is supposed to stimulate removal of accumulated waste, especially in joints. Powdered root (30-60 grains) has been used as an expectorant and diaphoretic.

Toxicity: Not much is known about its toxicity. Few cases have been recorded. Large doses do produce nausea, vomiting, and diarrhea, which is typical of most saponins. Hemolysis may occur in large doses, but this has not been shown.

Comments: There does not appear to be any basis for its use for rheumatism or biliary colic.

References: 2, 17, 36

Rhubarb
(*Rheum officinalis* or *R. palmatum*)

Known Principles: The plant contains anthraquinone derivatives of emodin, chrysophanol, aloe-emodin, and tannins. It yields not less than 35% alcohols.

Mode of Action: This product has both astringent and anthraquinone purgative properties. The anthraquinones are strong stimulant cathartics. With low doses, the astringent effects predominate over the cathartic actions.

Alleged Uses: The bark is dried and used in doses of 0.2–1 gm. In small doses its astringency is used against diarrhea. Larger amounts *cause* diarrhea.

Toxicity: The product may be a severe purgative. Cramping and severe fluid loss might occur. Safer and less drastic purgatives are available.

Comments: This is *not* the common garden rhubarb, which is *Rheum rhaponticum*. Garden rhubarb is not a strong cathartic.

References: 1, 3, 7, 8, 29

Rose
(*Rosa* spp.)

Known Principles: Most rose hips are high in vitamins A and C. The leaves contain tannins as well. Some members of this family have cyanogenic glycosides in the leaves. The petals have astringents, quercitrin, volatile oils, and colors comprised of anthocyanins and cyanins (10%).

Mode of Action: Most of rose's pharmacologic actions are due to its astringent and antiscorbutic properties.

Alleged Uses: Indians have used the leaves as a potherb, eaten the fruits as a nutrient, made leaves and petals into tea and salads, or candied them. The roots have been used in teas or smoked like tobacco.

Toxicity: Roses are almost always nontoxic. Large amounts may give diarrhea. The cyanogenic glycosides would only rarely present a problem.

References: 2, 3, 12, 17, 23, 26, 29

Rosemary
(Rosmarinus officinalis)

Known Principles: Rosemary contains approximately 1% volatile oil containing d-pinene, camphene, cineole, borneol (10–15%), 2–6% esters (bornyl acetate), and camphor. There are also a resin and a bitter principle.

Mode of Action: Most of rosemary's activity is related to the irritating properties of its volatile oil.

Alleged Uses: Rosemary has been used as a carminative, emmenagogue, and as a rubefacient in liniment. Nonmedically, it is used as both a condiment and as an ingredient in perfumes, hair lotions, and soaps.

Toxicity: There are no cited cases of serious poisoning by rosemary. All volatile oils are irritating; therefore, nausea and vomiting are possible with this herb. Since so little data are available, care should be taken when using this plant medicinally.

References: 9, 17

Rue
(Ruta graveolens)

Known Principles: Rue contains 0.1% of a greenish or yellow volatile oil contained in the glandular hairs on the aerial surfaces of the plant. This oil is 90% methyl-nonyl-ketone, with some other ketones, esters, and phenols. Rue also contains a bitter principle and the glycoside rutin. Leaves have been shown to contain both a volatile oil and tannins.

Mode of Action: The volatile oil is irritating. When applied to the skin it causes burning, redness, and vesiculation. Internally it may cause violent gastric pain, vomiting, prostration, confusion, and abortion in pregnant women. Some studies have shown that its stimulant action on uterine muscle is weak; however, in large doses, rutin will prolong the action of epinephrine and decrease capillary permeability.

Alleged Uses: Leaves have a strong, disagreeable odor, especially when rubbed. The taste is bitter, hot, and acrid. Rue is currently recommended for hysteria, worms, colic, and as an antispasmodic and uterine stimulant. It has found some use in Europe for criminal abortions. Fresh leaves may inflame or blister the skin and this plant is known to cause dermatitis.

Toxicity: Besides inducing various types of skin rashes, this plant has been known to produce kidney irritation and degeneration of the liver. Abortions due to this plant are more a result of general toxicity than of actual stimulation of the uterus. Large doses when taken internally cause violent gastric pains, vomiting, and prostration.

References: 1, 3, 7, 16

Saffron
(*Crocus sativus*)

Known Principles: Saffron contains two glycosides and a volatile oil.

Mode of Action: Little is known concerning these two glycosides or the volatile oil. As yet, no mechanism of action has been postulated for either its therapeutic or toxic effects.

Alleged Uses: The flowers are used to prepare both a drug and coloring agent. It has been used as a respiratory stimulant in asthma, tuberculosis, and whooping cough, as well as an abortifacient. It is also thought to be an aphrodisiac. Normal doses given range from 0.6–2 gms.

Toxicity: Chief toxic symptoms include flushing, epistaxis, vertigo, vomiting, bradycardia, and stupor. Fatalities have been reported when the drug has been used as an abortifacient.

References: 3, 4, 5, 6, 7, 16, 17

Sage
(*Salvia officinalis*)

Known Principles: Besides a resin, tannins, and a bitter principle, there is 1–2.5% volatile oil. This oil is composed of a terpene, thujone, camphor, and salvene. The fresh oil has the highest concentration of the terpene, but if left standing, the thujone and camphor predominate.

Mode of Action: Sage's antisecretory action is presumably a central function of the volatile oil. Sage has also been accredited with antispasmodic, antibacterial, and fever-reducing action. The mechanisms for these functions are not known. The carminative action is most likely due to the irritating effects of the volatile oil.

Alleged Uses: Sage is used nonmedically as a flavoring agent, insect repellant, and perfume. Medically it is used more frequently in Europe than the U.S. to decrease secretions (especially salivation), to decrease spasms, and as a carminative in colds and coughs. The dose used is 1.3–4 gms of powdered sage.

Toxicity: Garden sage is not highly toxic. Excessive amounts may cause dry mouth or local irritation. Little is known about its toxic effects.

Comments: *Salvia* is *not* red sage, or the brush sage of the desert. These are different plants with different properties and toxicities.

References: 1, 9, 17

Sarsaparilla
(Smilax aristolochiaefolis, S. regelii, S. febrifuga, S. ornata)

Known Principles: Besides containing a resin, volatile oil, starch, and calcium oxalates, sarsaparilla also contains sarsasapogenin, which is the sapogenin of sarsaponin; smilagenin (isosarsasapogenin), and other phytosterols (sitosterol, stigmasterol). The parillin and smilagin that have previously been reported are, in fact, impure forms of sarsasaponin.

Mode of Action: Besides the irritant actions of saponins, sarsaparilla has been shown to have hemolytic action. This was once proposed as an assay method for this drug.

Alleged Uses: Sarsaparilla root has a sweetish taste and mucilaginous feel. It is used as a pharmaceutical necessity and as a flavoring agent. The torn bark from the stem has been applied to the teeth for toothache, and it has even been recommended to increase sexual potency. In the Middle East, sarsaparilla has been used with dapsone in the treatment of leprosy. This plant was used against syphilis prior to 1757. The mechanism for its action against syphilis is unknown. Hot infusions of sarsaparilla

have been used against psoriasis. Commercial sarsaparilla is likely to be nearly inert due to either age or
inferior species included in the commercial mix. If the
leaves leave an acrid taste after chewing for a few minutes, the quality of the sarsaparilla is good. Normal dose
internally is 2–4 gms.

Toxicity: There have not been many recorded cases of sarsaparilla toxicity. There appears to be little danger. The
berries are listed as edible.

References: 2, 3, 16, 17, 24

Sassafras
(Sassafrass albidum)

Known Principles: Sassafras yields not less than 4 mls of volatile oil from each 100 gms of crude herb. Sassafras oil is
approximately 50% safrol, 10% pinene and phennan-
drene, 6–8% d-camphor, 0.5% eugenol, and 3%
cadinene.

Mode of Action: Volatile oils are mucous membrane irritants
and CNS depressants. These effects are possible.

Alleged Uses: The root bark is used as a hot infusion for
colds. Since it is less of a mucous membrane irritant than
other volatile oils, it is a less powerful carminative. It possesses considerable antiseptic power due to phenolic
properties.

Toxicity: The oil may be toxic, causing nausea, vomiting,
dilated pupils, cardiovascular collapse, and CNS depression. The safrol component of the oil causes respiratory
paralysis, and fatty degeneration of heart, liver, and kidneys. As little as 5 mls of oil can be seriously toxic in an adult.

Comments: The concentration of oil in the root is low, but use of more than 100 gms at one time may cause acute poisoning.

References: 17

Saw Palmetto Berries
(*Serenoa repens*) (Sabal)

Known Principles: The most evident ingredient in saw palmetto berries is 1.5% oil, composed of 60% free fatty acids, and 40% ethyl esters of these acids. These fatty acids are caproic, caprylic, capric, lauric, palmitic, and oleic. Some report a volatile oil as well, but it may be a degradation product of the fatty acid oil. There doesn't appear to be any alkaloid, but both a resin and a sugar have been reported.

Mode of Action: The pharmacology of this agent is not well understood. Some of these fatty acids are irritants to the mucous membranes and this may account for some of their recommended uses.

Alleged Uses: Saw palmetto finds its greatest use in treating chronic cystitis and serving as a mucous membrane stimulant to the genitourinary tract. It has effects similar to cubeb. Patients claim it gives relief of pain caused by irritation of bladder and urethra. The berries are said to be edible but not good. Normal dose is 0.65 to 1.3 gms.

Toxicity: Large amounts might cause diarrhea. There are no reports of serious toxicity.

References: 2, 9, 17, 26

Scotch Broom
(*Cytisus scoparius*)

Known Principles: In 1918, Valeur reported two alkaloids besides the 0.25–1% sparteine that had been discovered before. One is a nonvolatile called sarothamnine, the other a volatile called genisteine. There is also a glycoside called scaparin (1937), and hydroxytyramine. The maximum alkaloid content occurs in May and then decreases in June. Cytisine may also be present.

Mode of Action: Sparteine sulfate has been used as an oxytocic, and the effect of genisteine is similar to, but weaker than, sparteine. The action of the whole plant is quite different from either of these principles. Some studies have shown the scaparin to have a weak diuretic action, but it is most likely physiologically inert. Certain of the plant extracts will produce a sharp rise in blood pressure—most likely caused by the hydroxytyramine.

Alleged Uses: The whole plant has a bitter, nauseous taste and strong odor when bruised. The part of the plant used is the tops of branches from the shrub. It has been used in dropsy, but is now almost out of this use. Scotch broom is also recommended as a diuretic, cathartic, and as an emetic in large doses. Recently it has been recommended the plant be smoked to produce a sedative-hypnotic effect.

Toxicity: Human poisonings are rare; some have been reported in livestock in Europe. At a minimum, large doses should cause prolonged vomiting.

Comments: Scotch broom was formerly recognized by both the USP and NF.

References: 1, 3, 11, 17, 22, 29, 30

Scullcap
(Scutellaria lateriflora)

Known Principles: The active ingredients of scullcap include a volatile oil (scutellarin), a bitter glycoside, tannins, fat, sugar, and cellulose.

Mode of Action: The usual irritant effects of volatile oils are possible, but scullcap produces no obvious effects when taken internally in "therapeutic" amounts.

Alleged Uses: The whole plant is used to prepare a tonic that is usually used as an antispasmodic. The dose is ½–1 teaspoonful of the tonic.

Toxicity: One reference stated overdose produces giddiness, stupor, confusion, hyperreflexia, irregular pulse, and CNS stimulation. This information is confusing in view of the low pharmacologic activity of this agent. More study is needed.

References: 5, 6, 7, 17

Serpentaria
(Aristolochia serpentaria) (Virginia Snakeroot)

Known Principles: Virginia snakeroot contains the bitter principle serpentaria, and 0.5–2% volatile oil. The bitter may be alkaloidal, but it is unknown. Other *Aristolochia* species do not contain poisonous alkaloids. The volatile oil is 60% esters of borneol, 40% terpene, and a bluish-green fluorescent oil.

Mode of Action: In moderate doses it acts as a gastric stimulant, possible by its bitter taste. As a moderate stimulant, it is of some use in atonic types of dyspepsia.

Alleged Uses: Herbalists claim that serpentaria will increase circulation and stimulate the heart and mucous membranes. It is a bitter that is often recommended for dyspepsia. The dried roots and rhizomes are made into teas and tinctures that are recommended for fevers, smallpox, pneumonia, and skin sores. Normal dose of the tincture is 1–20 drops.

Toxicity: The herb is a local irritant. Symptoms that may occur include nausea, vomiting, griping pain, and tenesmus. Some of the alkaloids have caused death in animals.

Comments: Be sure of the genus and species name when dealing with snakeroot. There are many different plants with this common name.

References: 1, 2, 17, 36, 39

Silverwood
(*Potentilla answerina*) (Goose-tansy)

Known Principles: The primary ingredients appear to be tannins and small amounts of other organic acids such as kinovic and ellagic acid.

Mode of Action: Tannins are astringents and protein precipitants. A 1942 study showed that silverweed has a stimulant action on animal uterine muscle; therefore, it may be of some use in dysmenorrhea.

Alleged Uses: The powdered weed is often used in combination with lobelia to treat tetanus when a physician is not available. Dose for this is 15–40 drops of the tincture.

Toxicity: There have been no reports of toxicity, although tannic acid could be a gastrointestinal irritant and renal toxin.

Comments: This herb does not appear to be active in areas related to tetanus.

References: 3, 17, 36

Slippery Elm
(*Ulmus fulva*)

Known Principles: Elm contains a polysaccharide, a mucilage similar to linseed, and small amounts of starch, tannins, calcium oxalate, and calcium.

Mode of Action: The mucilage acts as a demulcent.

Alleged Uses: The bark has been used in poultices for inflamed wounds and skin diseases, as well as an expectorant and gastrointestinal demulcent.

Toxicity: Toxic ingestions have not been reported but the plant may cause skin rashes.

References: 3, 4, 5, 6

Snakeroot
(*Rauwolfia serpentina*)

Known Principles: This herb contains reserpine, along with 5–20 other alkaloids, including yohimbine, serpentine, serpentinine, and amajaline.

Mode of Action: Reserpine has both a sedative and hypotensive effect. It is not a narcotic or hypnotic but causes its depression by depleting catecholamines and serotonin from both central and peripheral nerve fibers.

Alleged Uses: *Rauwolfia* has been recommended for a myriad of uses for centuries. The people of India think it is useful for all types of nervous disorders as a purgative, anthelmintic, and antidote for snake or insect bites. Its primary medical use currently is as a sedative and hypotensive agent.

Toxicity: Serious symptoms of toxicity can occur with 25–260 mg of reserpine. The actual lethal dose on a mg/kg basis has not yet been determined. Most poisonings occur in children. Symptoms include drowsiness, stupor, nasal congestion, diarrhea, intense gastric acid secretion, pinpoint pupils, hypotension, bradycardia, and decreased temperature.

Comments: Recent animal studies indicate that reserpine may be carcinogenic.

References: 2, 3, 9, 17, 22, 46

Spanish Broom
(*Spartium junceum*)

Known Principles: In 1927 the flowers were found to contain the alkaloid sparteine, but cytisine along with methylcystinine and anagyrine are considered the principle alkaloids.

Mode of Action: Sparteine sulfate (Spartocin™) has been employed as an oxytoxic. (Usual dose for labor induction

was 75 mg intravenously.) Cytisine is a quinolizidine alkaloid similar to nicotine in its actions.

Alleged Uses: As with Scotch broom, it is used primarily as a
diuretic, cathartic, and emetic. It is considered to be more
potent than Scotch broom. Dose of the seeds is 0.6–1 gm.

Toxicity: Poisonings have resulted in accidentally using
Spanish broom in place of Scotch broom. Symptoms expected would include nausea, vomiting, and diarrhea.
Renal damage is also possible, as would be the muscle-
paralyzing effects common to quinolizidine alkaloids.

Comments: Do not confuse with Scotch broom.

References: 17, 29

Spearmint
(Mentha spicata)

Known Principles: Spearmint contains resins, tannins, and a
volatile oil composed of approximately 50% carvone (a
ketone).

Mode of Action: The flavor is due to the volatile oil. The oil's
irritating aspects is most likely why it has found use as a
carminative.

Alleged Uses: Spearmint is used primarily as a flavor and
carminative. It has a warm and slightly bitter taste. Dose
of plant material is approximately 4 gms.

Toxicity: The dried plant material itself is not likely to be
very toxic. Children have become poisoned on as little as
5–10 ml of various volatile oils: therefore much care
should be taken when the oil is used instead of the dried
plant material. Symptoms include gastrointestinal irrita-

tion and central nervous system depression or stimulation, depending on the amounts ingested.

Comments: Spearmint has been recognized in official compendia since 1820.

References: 1, 3, 9, 17

Spirea
(*Filipendula ulmaria*)

Known Principles: Spirea contains a colorless volatile oil composed mainly of salicylic aldehyde with small amounts of methyl salicylate. Spiroaic acid (salicylic acid) was separated from the flowers. When fresh, the roots contain some volatile oils; they also have some tannic acid and gallic acid.

Mode of Action: The tannins and acids would be astringents and therefore mildly useful in treating diarrhea. The reason for its purported diuretic action is unknown. There may be some analgesic effect from the salicylate.

Alleged Uses: Decoctions of flowers are used as a diuretic. Roots are astringent and have been used against diarrhea. The dose of an aqueous extract of the root is 0.3–1.3 grams.

Toxicity: There is no evidence of toxic ingestions with this plant. Large amounts could cause salicylate poisoning or kidney damage from tannins.

Comments: Aspirin (acetylsalicylic acid) was named "a" from acetyl and "spirin" from spirea, the original source of salicylic acid.

References: 2, 3, 17

St. John's Wort
(*Hypericum perforatum*)

Known Principles: The ingredients include a volatile oil, a resin, a tannin, and a dye called hypericin.

Mode of Action: The dye has been documented to produce photosensitization in cattle who eat the plant. It is also reported to be an antidepressant in humans.

Alleged Uses: Although claimed to be of use in a wide variety of both internal and external complaints, it has fallen into disuse. One of its primary recommended uses by herbalists was as a cure for demonics.

Toxicity: The plant seems to be relatively safe in humans but care should be taken due to its photosensitizing abilities.

References: 17

Strawberry
(*Fragaria vesa, F. americana, F.* spp.)
(Earth Mulberry)

Known Principles: Strawberry leaves are known to contain vitamin C, minerals, catechins, and leucoanthocyanin.

Mode of Action: The ascorbic acid (vitamin C) is both astringent and antiscorbutic. Catechins are protein precipitants and astringents. The d-catechin is thought to inhibit production of histamine. It has little therapeutic action on its own but seems to potentiate antihistamine drugs if used with them.

Alleged Uses: Berries are thought to be helpful in treating kidney stones, perhaps because of the acidity of vitamin C. Roots and leaves have been suggested for treatment of eczema, diarrhea, toothache, and skin ulcers. Most actions are related to acidity, astringency, or mineral content.

Comments: The wild strawberry is a member of the rose family.

References: 2, 12, 17, 23, 36, 39, 52

Sumac
(*Rhus glabra, R. blabrum*)

Known Principles: The fruit contains malic acid, tannins, fixed oil, and a small amount of volatile oil. The bark has a soft resin, a volatile principle, albumin, gum, and tannin.

Mode of Action: The bark is astringent and mildly antiseptic, while the berries are a refrigerant and diuretic.

Alleged Uses: Sumac has been a domestic remedy used for its astringent and antiseptic properties. It has been recommended for dysentery, rectal hemorrhages, and various other rectal conditions. Leaves have even been smoked as a treatment for asthma.

Toxicity: There is very little information that would allow one to think of sumac as toxic. It does not have the strong irritants like other members of the *Rhus* family, i.e. poison ivy, poison oak.

References: 1, 2, 3, 9, 17, 36

Sundew
(Drosea rotundifolia)

Known Principles: *Drosea* is known to contain a resin, malic acid, citric acid, tannin, and droserone (2-methyl-5-hydroxy-1, 4, naphthoquinone).

Mode of Action: Other than having an acidic taste, it is thought to be inert.

Alleged Uses: Herbalists claim that it is an effective remedy for whooping cough, laryngitis, and smokers' cough.

Toxicity: There are no toxic ingestions noted. It is not considered toxic.

Comments: There is no basis in fact for its claim as a cough remedy.

References: 1, 2, 3, 9, 17, 36

Sunflower
(Helianthus annuus)

Known Principles: The primary ingredients are a yellow dye and a fixed oil. This oil consists of palmitic acid 6.4%, stearic acid 1.3%, arachidic acid 4%, behenic acid 0.8%, oleic acid 21.3%, linoleic acid 66.2%, and linolenic acid less than 0.1%. The oil is defined as a semidrying oil of the oleic-linoleic acid type. The seeds contain 75 mg/100 grams of vitamin E.

Mode of Action: Experimentally, sunflowers have shown a small amount of blood sugar-reducing ability. It is not used medically this way, however. The oil is used as a food source and to treat fatty acid deficiency. Little else has been said about the specific actions of the fatty acids in the oil, or what other chemicals may be in the leaves and flowers to produce the professed effects.

Alleged Uses: Tinctures of the leaves and flowers have been combined with balsamic drugs for the treatment of bronchial inflammations and cold. Peoples of the Caucasus use the leaves to treat malarial fevers. Dazel, in 1920, did a study that seemed to indicate it was useful in this regard, but no active principle was isolated. At one time, individuals made an infusion that was used to kill flies. Pioneers placed green or dried flowers in a warm bath for the relief of rheumatism. (Whether it was the sunflowers or the warm water that gave the relief is hard to ascertain.) The seeds are claimed to increase urine flow and sweating. Sunflowers have many uses; the stems yield a fine textile fiber, the leaves are used for fodder, and the seeds and oil are consumed as a food.

Toxicity: There seems to be very little toxicity. If grown in a high nitrate area, they could accumulate these chemicals but it is seldom a significant problem.

References: 1, 3, 9, 17, 39, 52

Sweet Violet
(Viola odorata, V. pedapa)

Known Principles: Sweet violet is said to contain myrosin and several other unidentified glycosides.

Mode of Action: As far back as 500 B.C., violets have been recommended as a poultice for surface cancer. In the 18th century, the medical literature again recommended violets for the treatment of cancers. One 1960 experiment done on cancerous mice did show that a violet extract caused damage to cancers harbored by the mice. There has been little experimentation since this to further substantiate antineoplastic activity, or to indicate what in violet may produce these effects.

Alleged Uses: Sweet violet has been recommended by herbalists for a number of uses. These include treatment for skin diseases, a mild laxative, to induce vomiting, as an expectorant, and as an aid in controlling the cough of whooping cough, especially when accompanied by shortness of breath.

Toxicity: The flowers and seeds of the violet are reported to be edible. The seed, however, may produce a dramatic cathartic effect.

Comments: More research needs to be done on sweet violet before any conclusions can be drawn on its activity. At this point, it does appear to have some mucous membrane irritant effects that may cause catharsis or provide it with an expectorant action. There may also be some antineoplastic activity.

References: 3, 36, 39, 43

Tansy
(Tanacetum vulgare)

Known Principles: The flowers of tansy contain three resins, a bitter principle, and the volatile oil tanacetone. This oil has been found to be identical to thujone with small amounts of camphor and borneol.

Mode of Action: The oil does seem to be effective against roundworms. Although one study showed it does not appear to have a stimulant effect on the uterus, it has caused abortion in cattle. Thujone was shown to be a uterine stimulant in animals (all studies).

Alleged Uses: Considered by herbalists to be an irritant and narcotic, it is used as a vermifuge, as a treatment for amenorrhea and dysmenorrhea, and to produce abortions. The flowers, seeds, and leaves are all used to produce various beverages with an extremely bitter, warm taste.

Toxicity: There have been several fatalities caused by this herb in both humans and animals. As little as 4 mls of the oil have caused death. Symptoms usually seen include nausea, vomiting, dilated pupils, weak and fast pulse, coma, convulsions, and even death.

Comments: This is a dangerous herb and should be used only with medical supervision.

References: 2, 11, 17, 36

Thunder God Vine
(*Tripterygium wilfordii*) (Lei Kung Teng)

Known Principles: The primary compound is an alkaloidal substance called wilfordine. Wilfordine is actually a combination of several alkaloids such as wilforine, wilfordine, wilforgine, wilfortine, and wilforzine. There are also triptolide and tripdiolide in the plant.

Mode of Action: Wilfordine is insecticidal. Triptolide and tripdiolide may have some antineoplastic activity.

Alleged Uses: This plant is usually applied externally or left surrounding an area to be protected from insects. There are no reports of it being used internally.

Toxicity: There are no reports of toxicity, but data are very limited. Caution should be taken with any plant containing this many alkaloids.

References: 16, 17

Thyme
(*Thymus vulgaris*)

Known Principles: The ingredients most commonly mentioned are thyme oil, tannins, and gum.

Mode of Action: The phenols in the oil may be responsible for its antiseptic activity. It also possesses a carminative action like most volatile oil.

Alleged Uses: The dried leaves and flowering tops are used as a carminative and antiseptic. It has been recommended widely for cough, bronchitis, and a treatment for hookworm. There is only a small margin of safety when thyme is used to treat hookworm.

Toxicity: Large doses of thyme oil result in a phenol-like poisoning. Doses of 0.2–1 ml of pure oil have been reported to cause poisoning.

References: 1, 3, 4, 5, 6, 16, 17

Tonka Bean
(*Coumarouna odorata, Dipteryx odorta*)
(Tonquin Bean)

Known Principles: Although tonka bean contains 25% fixed oil, starch, sitosterin, stigmasterin, sugar, and gum, the primary active ingredient is 1–10% coumarin.

Mode of Action: Coumarin is a anticoagulant. It interferes with the synthesis of vitamin K-dependent clotting factors, preventing adequate blood clotting.

Alleged Uses: The seeds are pulverized, then treated to release the coumarin. They have a strong agreeable odor and a bitter, aromatic taste. For some time the beans were used as a flavor until the FDA banned it as a food additive. It is still used as a flavoring for some tobacco.

Toxicity: The coumarin is a potentially dangerous compound. As little as 50 mg/kg of coumarin can be fatal for animals. For the average human, this would work out to about 100 mgs (¼ lb.) of beans, assuming the concentration of coumarin to be about 3.5%. When animals have been fed this compound regularly, it causes extensive liver damage, growth retardation, and testicular atrophy.

Comments: Tonka beans were at one time a common adulterate in vanilla. Besides its toxicity, coumarin interacts with a number of drugs and should be used only on the advice of a physician.

References: 2, 17, 21, 51

Tormentil
(Potentilla erecta, P. tormentil)

Known Principles: This plant contains a red coloring principle that appears to be identical to rhatany-red, 10–15% tannins, and small amounts of kinovic and ellagic acid.

Mode of Action: The plant's primary action is as a powerful astringent.

Alleged Uses: The roots are a moderate to powerful astringent used to treat dysentery, sore throat, and in a poultice for wounds. Some claim that it is a remedy for venereal diseases like gonorrhea.

Toxicity: Very little is available regarding its toxicity. The 10–15% tannins could produce gastritis and even renal damage if taken in significant amounts.

References: 1, 2, 17, 36, 39

Valerian Root
(Valeriana edulis, V. officinalis)
(Garden Heliotrope)

Known Principles: The plant contains several alkaloids and glycosides, as well as several resinous bodies, and a brown-yellow volatile oil. The total alkaloid content is approximately 0.1% and is composed of primarily chatinine and valerine. The volatile oil consists of formic, acetic, butyric, and valeric acid esters of borneol, as well as pinene and camphene. Exposure to air causes decomposition of the oil.

Mode of Action: This plant may produce a slight central nervous system depressant effect; however, the exact activity and mechanism are not resolved. This action is usually lost upon drying the plant. The depressant effect is most likely due to the alkaloids and glycosides, but it also has a ketone and volatile oil that will produce this effect. Which agent actually gives the depression is not yet understood.

Alleged Uses: This powdered root is most often prepared as a fluid extract with a disagreeable odor. Although valerian's physiological actions are weak, it does have some central nervous system depressant activity that has led to its use as a tranquilizer for treatment of hysteria, hypochondriasis, nervous unrest, insomnia, and convulsion. Many think its primary effect now is a psychologic rather than a physiologic one. Indians thought the raw roots were poisonous, so they usually cooked them before eating. It has a very strong, disagreeeable odor.

Toxicity: Serious overdoses have not been reported, but with so many constituents, sufficient quantities are bound to produce vomiting and drowsiness. Usual amounts do not represent a serious hazard.

Comments: Cats seem to be attracted to this herb.

References: 1, 3, 4, 5, 6, 12, 17, 22

Watercress
(Nasturtium officinale)

Known Principles: This herb is known to contain significant amounts of vitamins A, C, B$_1$, and B$_2$, and to be rich in minerals.

Mode of Action: Large amounts of vitamin C could acidify the urine and possibly decrease the size of some types of bladder or urethral stones. The difficulty in assuming this is that acidic urine may create or worsen other types of stones. Also, a large amount of watercress would need to be ingested to produce this effect. The plant is antiscorbutic, of course, and a good source of vitamins and minerals.

Alleged Uses: Besides its recommendation as a fine potherb, watercress is many times used to treat various kidney ailments and to increase urine flow. Other recommendations include treatment for heart trouble, ease of labor pain, or treatment for tuberculosis. There is little basis for any of these claims.

Toxicity: Unless this herb is mistaken for another plant like water hemlock, there is little evidence that it is toxic.

References: 36, 39, 52

White Cohosh
(*Actaea alba, A. arguta*)

Known Principles: Active constituents are not well established but thought to be glycosides or an essential oil. Protoanemonin is thought to be the irritant substance.

Mode of Action: Little is known, but the protoanemonin is a strong mucous membrane irritant and may be toxic.

Alleged Uses: Herbalists use white cohosh as a "woman's remedy," sedative, and dependable emmenagogue. Dose is 2–5 drops of the tincture.

Toxicity: All parts of the plant are toxic, producing skin rashes and eye irritation externally, and severe gastritis, bloody diarrhea, and possible hallucinations internally. Symptoms usually occur within 30 minutes of an ingestion and last about an hour.

Comments: The plant appears too dangerous to use for the nonspecific illness listed and may cause serious harm.

References: 3, 36

White Pine
(Pinus strobus, P. alba)

Known Principles: Besides approximately 10% tannic acid, an oleoresin, a volatile oil, coniferyl alcohol, and considerable mucilage, there is a small amount of coniferin. Coniferin, when hydrolyzed and then oxidized, is converted to vanillin.

Mode of Action: The coniferin is probably not of any therapeutic value. Medicinal action is more likely to lie with the volatile oil or the resin, both of which are mild expectorants.

Alleged Uses: The plant part used as a pharmaceutical necessity is the inner layer of bark. The usual dose is approximately 1–3 gms. Its taste is bitter and astringent. Since white pine is most often used in combination with other expectorants for cough syrups, it is difficult to assess whether it has any real therapeutic value. The coniferin is sometimes extracted and used as a commercial source of vanillin.

Toxicity: There are no reports of serious poisoning with this herb.

References: 9, 17

Wild Hyssop

(Verbena officinalis) (European Vervaine)

Known Principles: Vervaine contains the iridoid glycoside verbenaline, which is said to be equivalent to the glycoside cornin.

Mode of Action: Specific information concerning the action of verbenaline is limited. This glycoside is very bitter and is said to have some nauseating power, creating vomiting in mild to moderate doses. It also has some weak stimulant effect upon parasympathetic nerves. Some of the iridoid glycosides are external antibacterials.

Alleged Uses: Wild hyssop has for a long time been a family remedy for whooping cough, stomachache, or for induction of vomiting. Any part of the plant may be used, but the root portion makes a stronger tincture. The normal recommended dose by herbalists is 20–40 drops in water taken as needed.

Toxicity: The alkaloid verbenaline is said to be low in toxicity and is nonhemolytic. Specific information on nontoxic exposures to vervaine is absent. Since this herb contains an active emetic, care should be taken that excessive amounts are not used, or severe gastritis may occur.

References: 1, 17, 36, 37, 39

Wild Lettuce

(Lactuca virosa, L. sativa, or *L. scariola)*

Known Principles: *Lactuca* contains a milky juice made up of 0.2% lactucin, 50% lactucerol, and latucic acid, caoutchouc, a volatile oil, and mannite. Some references also report the presence of hyoscyamine, but this is not well documented at this time. There also appears to be a high concentration of nitrates.

Mode of Action: There are no real pharmacologic data to substantiate use as a narcotic. The presence of hyoscyamine would lend credence to its depressant claims.

Alleged Uses: Its most common recommended use is as a sedative, usually in cough medication as a substitute for opium. Occasionally it has been recommended in the treatment of angina pectoris. One of its current uses involves smoking it for its "high " effect.

Toxicity: Wild lettuce appears to be quite low in toxicity. The only poisoning cases involve cattle who developed pulmonary emphysema, severe dyspnea, and weakness after eating the immature plants of *L. scariola.* Postmortem finding showed destruction of lung tissue. Only the immature plants appear toxic. Since the animals needed to eat large amounts, it is very unlikely that one would be poisoned by eating a small amount of the natural plant.

Comments: The plant's use as a "narcotic" is somewhat confusing, since it does not appear to have any activity and is quite an expensive herb. Perhaps just the title "lettuce opium" is enough to give it activity.

References: 3, 9, 17, 30

Wild Rue
(Peganum harmala) (African rue)

Known Principles: Wild rue contains 2.5–4% total alkaloids. The principle alkaloid is harmaline (60%) with harmine, harmalol, and peganine also present.

Mode of Action: These alkaloids have hallucinogenic properties. They have also been found to have antibacterial
and antiprotozoal activity.

Alleged Uses: Wild rue is used in India for various purposes,
but especially as an anthelmintic and narcotic. *Peganum* is
usually used in the form of an infusion or tincture.

Toxicity: Peganum may be hallucinogenic. This plant has
caused death in livestock and laboratory animals.
Symptoms of poisoning include posterior paralysis and
weakening of the voluntary muscles. Most symptoms appear within one hour of ingestion.

Comments: Wild rue may have an abuse potential in New
Mexico, Texas, and Arizona, where it is grown, because
of the possibility of hallucinogenic experiences while
using the plant.

References: 1, 11

Wintergreen
(*Gaultheria procumbens*)

Known Principles: Wintergreen contains a glycoside (mono-
tropitoside), which when hydrolyzed by an enzyme found
in the plant releases methyl salicylate.

Mode of Action: The methyl salicylate is a gastric irritant and
is likely to give stomach distress if taken by mouth. This
oil is absorbed through the skin. Its primary use is as an
analgesic and counterirritant.

Alleged Uses: The leaves, stems, and rhizomes contain
methyl salicylate, which can be obtained by stem distillation of crushed plant material. The leaves are often made

into an agreeable tea. The oil contains about 98% esters of methyl salicylate.

Toxicity: Methyl salicylate is quite toxic, but there have been no recorded cases of toxic ingestions of the plant material.

Comments: The leaves and berries have been used by Indians and as a survival food. Toxicity is unlikely to occur unless very large amounts of the plant material are ingested, or an extract of the oil prepared.

References: 3, 17, 24

Witch Hazel
(*Hamamelis virginiana*)

Known Principles: Witch hazel contains 2.3–9.5% tannins called hamamelitannin and a second tannin thought to be derived from gallic acid. Besides these tannins, there are hexose sugar, volatile oil, gallic acid, a bitter principle, and calcium oxalate.

Mode of Action: The tannins are protein precipitants with astringent and hemostatic properties.

Alleged Uses: Witch hazel is used as a mild astringent in ointments, solutions, and suppositories. Its most common use has been in the treatment of hemorrhoids. Although recommended as a sedative, this claim medically is unsubstantiated. Its astringency may be the reason for its use in diarrhea and gonorrhea.

Toxicity: Tannins are usually not absorbed to any appreciable effect. Doses of 1 gm will cause nausea, vomiting, or constipation leading to impaction. Liver damage is possible if the tannins are absorbed to any appreciable extent.

References: 1, 2, 10, 17

Woodruff
(Asperula odorata, Galium odoratum)
(Woodward herb)

Known Principles: This herb contains an essential oil, bitter principle, fatty oil, tannins, asperuloside, and coumarin.

Mode of Action: There seems to be little therapeutic virtue in anything but the essential oil, which is a carminative and mild expectorant.

Alleged Uses: Woodruff's primary uses are as a flavoring agent in May wine or as an ingredient in sachets. It is rarely recommended as an expectorant in chronic cough.

Toxicity: No reports of toxic ingestions are noted.

References: 3, 9

Wormwood
(Artemisia absinthium)

Known Principles: Contains absinthol, a volatile oil.

Mode of Action: The volatile oil is a CNS depressant, causing trembling, then stupor followed by convulsions.

Alleged Uses: The dried leaves and flowering tops have been used as a stomachic and sedative. It has been abused almost like alcohol, resulting in a clinical condition called absinthism. The dose of the entire wormwood is 1.3–2.6 gms or 0.06–0.12 mls of the oil.

Toxicity: As little as 15 mls of the volatile oil caused coma and convulsions in an adult. Combinations of this drug can be habit forming.

References: 17, 22

Yarrow
(Achillea millefolium)

Known Principles: Yarrow is reported to contain a volatile oil, an alkaloid, tannins, achilleine, achilleic acid, and the bitter caledivain.

Mode of Action: The mechanism is unknown, but the alkaloid reduces the clotting time in rabbits, the action lasting for about 45 minutes, without noticeable toxic aftereffects.

Alleged Uses: The flowering tops and leaves have been used primarily as a tea to induce drowsiness and as an aid in amenorrhea. The normal dose is 2-4 gms.

Toxicity: No toxic ingestions are reported in current literature.

References: 17, 20

Yellow Cedar
(Thuja occidentalis) (Arbor vitae)

Known Principles: Yellow cedar contains the volatile oil thujone, some tannins, fenchone, thujetic acid, and pinipirin.

Mode of Action: The action of the oils thujone and fenchone is similar to camphor. They are central nervous system and cardiac stimulants. A 1911 study found the oil does have a stimulant effect on isolated uterine muscle, similar to hydrastis. Thujone is an anthelmintic.

Alleged Uses: *Thuja* is most often recommended as a remedy for muscular aches and pains not due to arthritis. It has occasionally been tried on warts.

Toxicity: Ingestions of thujone, the portion of cedar leaf oil, may cause convulsions, decrease in blood pressure, coma, and death. There have been deaths when this oil was misused as an abortifacient.

Comments: Cedar leaf oil is described as not less than 60% ketone, calculated as thujone. This is a moderately dangerous herb that should be used under medical supervision and certainly not by pregnant women.

References: 2, 9, 11, 17, 36

Yellow Dock
(*Rumex crispus*)

Known Principles: Dock contains oxalate, most likely potassium oxalate.

Mode of Action: Oxalate crystals seem to do their damage by mechanically penetrating the tissue and creating a wound. When the crystal is broken by freezing or boiling repeatedly, little damage occurs. The kidney is especially susceptible to the mechanical damage since the crystals are concentrated there for excretion.

Alleged Uses: Used with other spring leaves in salads, yellow dock has a sweet-sour taste. It is used as a laxative as well.

Toxicity: Handling the leaves may give dermatitis. Symptoms occurring about 2–6 hours after ingestion include nausea, vomiting, and diarrhea, as well as some oral irritation. If significant amounts are ingested, renal damage may occur.

Comments: Since the plant is usually boiled before use, much of the danger of ingesting this plant may be averted by destruction of the crystals.

References: 3, 28

Yerba Santa
(Eriodictyon californicum) (Bear's Weed)

Known Principles: Yerba santa contains several flavones, pentatriacontane eriodicytyol (the aglycone of eriodictin), tannic acid, a bitter resin, formic acid, and a volatile oil.

Mode of Action: The resin of this herb absorbs many basic substances, and therefore will mask the taste of bitter drugs. The resin is specific and does not do the same for acidic compounds. The volatile oil has irritant properties that makes it useful as an expectorant.

Alleged Uses: Yerba santa's primary use is to mask the flavor of other bitter drugs. The Southwestern Indians used it as an expectorant for hay fever, and for treatment of hemorrhoids.

Toxicity: There have been no reports of serious toxicity with this herb. The volatile oil could be irritating to the mucous membranes of the gastrointestinal tract if a large amount were taken.

References: 2, 16, 17, 23

Yohimbe
(Corynanthe yohimbe)

Known Principles: Yohimbe contains the alkaloid yohimbine (also called quebrachine, aphrodine and corynine). Yohimbine is a harmine analog; therefore, hallucinogenic properties are possible.

Mode of Action: Yohimbine produces an alpha-adrenergic block of short duration. Central nervous system activity is much less than that with ergot alkaloids. It does not block the action of ephedrine on the heart. It has been recommended to decrease high blood pressure, but in fact may increase blood pressure. It has a local anesthetic action about equal to that of cocaine, but is longer lasting and more irritating. Moderate doses give vasodilation of skin and other mucous membranes, especially the sexual organs. This is an effect which is seen more in animals and is not a common finding with therapeutic doses in humans. Although a harmine analog, yohimbine does not have true hallucinogenic properties. It has been known to produce an anxiety syndrome in humans when given intravenously.

Alleged Uses: Yohimbe has been recommended as an aphrodisiac (evidence lacking to document this), as treatment for dysmenorrhea, as an antidiuretic, to aid in angina pectoris, and to decrease blood pressure. Other purposes for which it is used include treatment of impotence and arteriosclerosis and as a local anesthetic. It has also been smoked or used in tea as an hallucinogen. Currently it is advertised as a smoking preparation for "effortless seduction." A dose is 2.5–5 mgs, up to three times a day.

Toxicity: Symptoms of overdose include hypertension, abdominal distress, weakness, and fatigue. Large amounts produce general nervous stimulation to the point of paralysis. When this paralysis affects the respiratory muscles, death is due to cessation of breathing.

Comments: Should not be used in kidney or liver diseases.

References: 1, 16, 25, 26, 27, 30

Herbal References

Note: *This list of references is being continuously expanded for use in future editions, and is therefore not in alphabetical order.*

1. Blacow, N. W. *Martindale Extra Pharmacopoela*. 26th ed. London: Pharmaceutical Press, 1972.
2. Claus, E. P., and Tyler, V. E. *Pharmacognosy*. 5th ed. Philadelphia: Lea and Febiger, 1965.
3. Rumack, B. H., et al. *Poisindex*. February 1977. ed. Denver: Micromedex, Inc.
4. Allport, N. L. *The Chemistry and Pharmacy of Vegetable Drugs*. New York: Chemical Publishing Company, Inc., 1944.
5. Steinmetz, E. F. *Materia Medical Vegetabilis*. Amsterdam: Keizergracht 714, 1954.
6. Grieve, M. *A Modern Herbal*. New York: Hefner Publishing, 1959.
7. Lampe, K. F., and Fagerstrom, R. *Plant Toxicity and Dermatitis*. Baltimore: Williams and Wilkins, 1968.
8. Hardin, J., and Arena, J. *Human Poisoning from Native and Cultivated Plants*. 2nd ed. Durham, N.C.: Duke University Press, 1974.
9. Stecher, P. *The Merck Index*. Rahway, N.J.: Merck and Co., 1968.
10. Kadans, J. M. *Modern Encyclopedia of Herbs*. West Nyack, N.Y.: Parker Publishing Co. 1974.
11. Kingsbury, J. M. *Poisonous Plants of the United States and Canada*. Englewood Cliffs, N.J.: Prentice-Hall, 1974.
12. Harrington, H. D. *Edible Native Plants of the Rocky Mountains*. Albuquerque: University of New Mexico Press, 1967.
13. Harris, B. C. *Eat the Weeds*. Barre, Mass.: Barre Publishers, 1968.
14. Gibbons, E. *Stalking the Healthful Herbs*. New York: David McKay Co., 1966.
15. Coon, N. *Using Plants for Healing*. Hearthside Press, 1963.
16. Lewis, W. H., Elvin, L.; and Memory, P. F. *Medical Botany*. New York· Wiley, 1977.

17. Osol, A., and Farrar, G. *The Dispensatory of the United States of America.* 25th ed. Philadelphia: J. P. Lippincott Co., 1975.
18. Jang, C. S. *Journal of Pharmacology,* 1941, 178.
19. Macht, D. I., and Cook, H. M. *J Am Pharm Ass,* 1932, 324.
20. Henry, T. *The Plant Alkaloids.* 4th ed. London: J. A. Churchill Ltd., 1949.
21. *Food and Drug Administration Compliance Policy Guides,* Chapter 17, Guide #7117.05, 77-21, March 1977.
22. Siegel, R. K. "Herbal Intoxication Problem," *JAMA* 236(5):473-76.
23. Der Marderosian, A. "Medicinal Teas—Boon or Bane?" *Drug Therapy,* February 1977.
24. Morton, J. F. *Herbs and Spices.* Racine, Wisc.: Golden Press, Western Publishing Co., 1976.
25. Farnsworth, N. R., and Bederda, J. P., Jr. *"Ginseng,"* Lilly Digest.
26. Arena, J. M. *Poisoning-Toxicology: Symptoms and Treatments.* 3rd. ed. Springfield, Ill.: Charles C. Thomas, 1976.
27. Gosselin, R. E.; Hodge, H. C.; Smith, R. P.; and Gleason, M. N. *Clinical Toxicology of Commercial Products.* 4th ed. Baltimore: Williams and Wilkins, 1976.
28. Lampe, K. F.; Hatfield, G. M.; and Snyder, D. S. "Harzardous Plants: The Calcium Oxalate Controversy." Paper presented at the meetings of the AAPCC, Chicago, Oct. 18-20, 1978.
29. Tyler, V. E.; Brady, L. R.; and Robbers, J. A. *Pharmacognosy.* 7th ed. Philadelphia: Lea and Febiger, 1976.
30. Brown, J. L., and Malone, M. H. "Legal Highs—Constituents, Activity, Toxicology, and Herbal Folklore," *Clinical Toxicology* 12(1):1-31.
31. Bryson, P. D.; Watanabe, A. S.; Rumack, B. H.; and Murphy, R. C. "Burdock Root Tea Poisoning—Case Report Involving a Commercial Preparation," *JAMA* 239:20.
32. Bouchey, G. D., and Gjerstad, G. "Chemical Studies of Aloe Vera Juice II,"*Quart J Crude Drug Res* 9(4):1445-53.
33. Cheney, R. H. "Aloe Drug in Human Therapy," *Quart J Crude Drug Res* 10(1):1523-30.
34. Medsger, O. P. *Edible Wild Plants.* New York: MacMillan, 1966.
35. "Back to Folk Medicine: The Pros and Cons," *Medical World News,* Dec. 7, 1973, pp. 65-68.
36. Clymer, R. S. *Nature's Healing Agents.* Quakertown, Pa.; The Humanitarian Society, 1973.
37. Wagner, H., and Wolff, P. *New Natural Products and Plant Drugs with Pharmacological, Biological or Therapeutical Activity.* Berlin: Springer-Verlag, 1977.

38. Altschul, S. R. *Drugs and Food From Little-Known Plants: Notes in Harvard University Herbaria.* Cambridge, Mass.: Harvard University Press, 1973.
39. Krochmal, A., and Krochmal, C. *A Guide to Medicinal Plants of the United States.* New York: Quadrangle/The New York Times Book Company, 1973.
40. Teteny, P. *Infraspecific Chemical Taxa of Medicinal Plants.* New York: Chemical Publishing Co., 1970.
41. Kreig, B. *Green Medicine, The Search For Plants That Heal.* Chicago: Rand McNally, 1964.
42. Sim, S. K. *Medicinal Plant Glycosides.* Toronto: University of Toronto Press, 1967.
43. Lucas, R. *Nature's Medicines.* West Nyack, N.Y.: Parker Publishing, 1966.
44. Dawson, R.; Landsburg, R.; and Riggs, J. *Edible Plant Cards of Temperate North America.* Manning, Oregon; Life Support Technology, 1975.
45. d'Andreta, C. *Herbs and Other Medicinal Plants.* New York: Crescent Books, 1972.
46. Emboden, W. *Narcotic Plants.* New York: MacMillan, 1972.
47. Lehner, E., and Lehner, J. *Folklore and Odyssey of Food and Medicinal Plants.* New York: Farrar, Straus, Giraux, 1973.
48. Stern, P., and Milin, R. "Die antiallergische und anti-phlogistische Wirkung der Azulene," *Arzneimittel-Forsch* 6:445-50.
49. Farnsworth, N., and Morgan, B. "Herb Drinks: Camomile Tea," *JAMA* 221:410.
50. Benner, B. H., and Lee, H. J. "Anaphylactic Reaction to Chamomile Tea," *J. Allergy Clin Immunol* 52:307-308.
51. Goodman, L. S., and Gilman, A. *The Pharmacological Basis of Therapeutics.* 5th ed. New York: MacMillan, 1975.
52. Angier, B. *Field Guide to Medical Wild Plants.* Harrisburg, Pa.: Stackpole Books, 1978.

Index